# My Way! No Way!

# TAO IS THE WAY!

## TAO Wisdom To Live And Survive
## In A World Of Depression

### STEPHEN LAU

## DEDICATION

This book is dedicated to those who have been struggling with depression. It is hoped that they will now use TAO wisdom to go *through* their depression and experience it in a totally new dimension.

# CONTENTS

# ACKNOWLEDGMENT

All the quotes from Lao Tzu are taken from the author's
book "The Complete Tao Te Ching in Plain English"
and all the Biblical quotes are from
the New International Version (NIV).

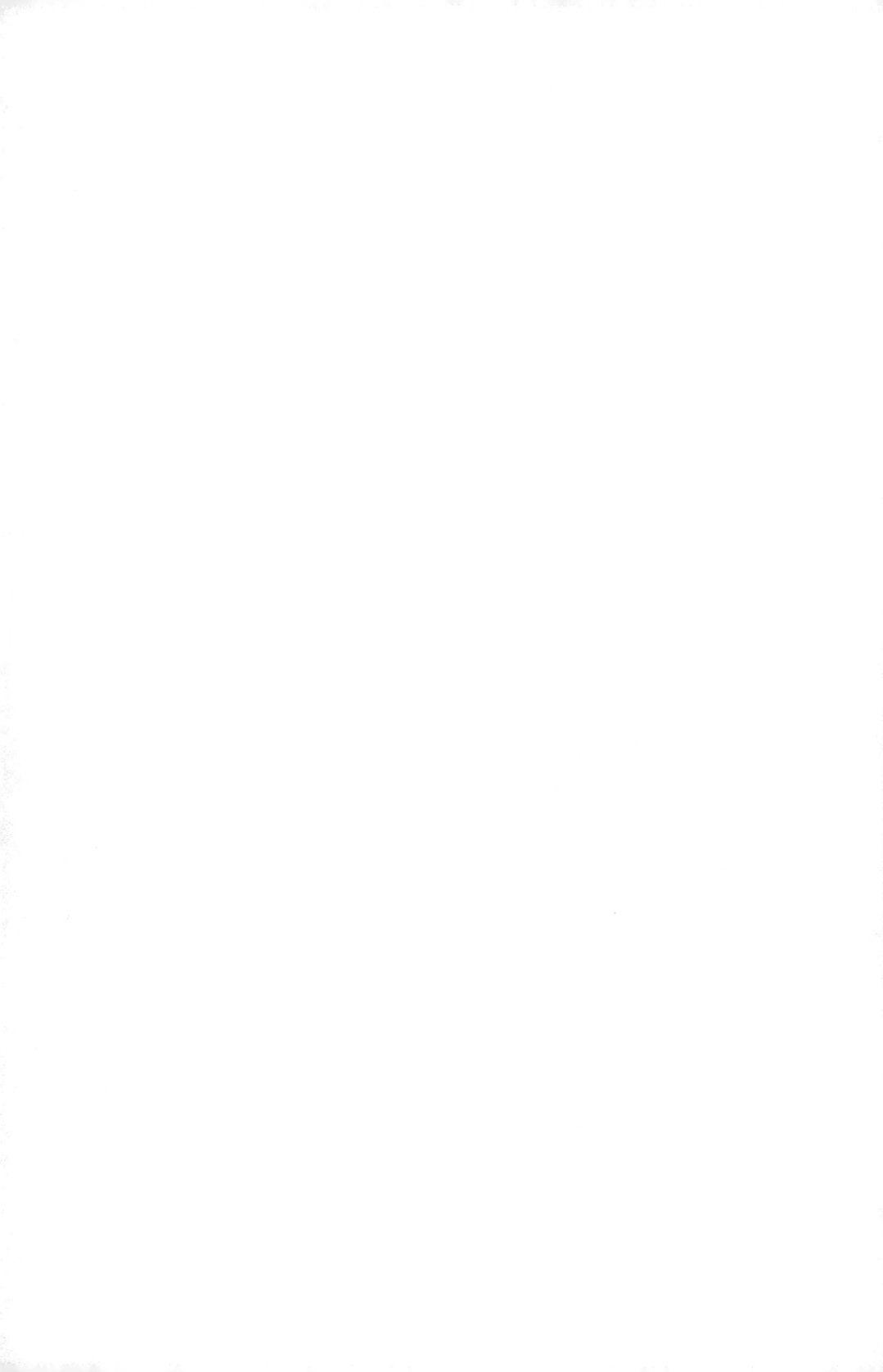

# INTRODUCTION

TAO is neither a religion nor a philosophy.

TAO is simply a way of life about the Way of life, that is, a general way of *thinking* about everything in life. It is a pathless path of humanity to live as if everything is a miracle.

TAO is the Way *through* anything and everything in life in order to fully experience them and live in balance and harmony. TAO is not about avoiding or getting out of anything unhappy and undesirable in everyday life, such as depression; rather, it is about going *through* depression by experiencing every aspect of it in order to become *enlightened*, if possible, with the profound human wisdom to continue living in peace and harmony in a world of depression.

TAO is looking at life not as a series of both happy and unhappy episodes, but simply as a journey of self-discovery and self-awakening to the real meaning of life existence. You are defined not by your words and thoughts, but by the ways you act and react, as well as the impact you may have on others around you. You exist not because you are simply here; you are here in this world to love and to learn how to live, as well as to help one another do the same.

TAO is formless, shapeless, and inexplicable in words; after all, it had existed long before there were even words. TAO is infinite human wisdom, which is a pathless path to the infinity and the origin of all things.

TAO is not about making your life any easier; it is about acceptance of all aspects of your humanity that need to be fully experienced, embraced, and then to be let go of in order to become wholesome at other times of your life and living—*that* is the essence of TAO wisdom, which is true enlightenment of the human mind.

Living in a world of depression, you might want everything your way or no way. But TAO *is* the Way *through* your depression, enabling you to understand *how* and *why* you might have your depression in the first place.

# ONE

# THE DEPRESSIVE MIND

## A World of Depression

"Depression has been called the world's number one public health problem. In fact, depression is so widespread it is considered the common cold of psychiatric disturbances. But there is a grim difference between depression and a cold. Depression can kill you." **David D. Burns**

We *all* have a depressive mind because we are all living in a world of depression. The only difference is that our depression may all differ in intensity: slight, serious, or severe. The truth of the matter is that each and every one of us *is* depressed, without any exception, because we *all* experience our depressive episodes at some points during our lifespan, and it is very *normal*. However, many of us prefer to deny or ignore our emotional dysfunction due to the stigma that is often associated with depression.

Depression is *not* a new human disease or disorder; it is as ancient as man:

so I have been allotted months of futility,
    and nights of misery have been assigned to me.

3

When I lie down I think, 'How long before I get up?'

The night drags on, and I toss and turn until dawn.

My body is clothed with worms and scabs,
my skin is broken and festering.

"My days are swifter than a weaver's shuttle,
and they come to an end without hope.

Remember, O God, that my life is but a breath;
my eyes will never see happiness again.

The eye that now sees me will see me no longer;
you will look for me, but I will be no more.

As a cloud vanishes and is gone,
so one who goes down to the grave does not return.

He will never come to his house again;
his place will know him no more.

"Therefore I will not keep silent;
I will speak out in the anguish of my spirit,
I will complain in the bitterness of my soul.

**(Job** 7: 3-11)

Answer me quickly, LORD; my spirit fails. Do not hide your face from me or I will be like those who go down to the pit. Let the morning bring me word of your unfailing love, for I have put my trust in you. Show me the way I should go, for to you I entrust my life.
**(Psalm** 143: 7-8)

In modern age, **Sir Winston Churchill**, the Prime Minister of Great Britain, underwent serious bouts of depression during his country's national crisis in World War II. The fact is that depression is no respecter of persons— even for those with very high I.Q., such as the Nobel Prize winning author **Ernest Hemingway** who committed suicide just as his father did with the comment "I'll probably go the same way." Indeed, many of us are vulnerable to this genetic mental disorder.

Sadly, depression is currently increasing at an alarming rate because the world we are now living in is getting more challenging, more complex, and more complicated each day passing—it has now become a world of depression.

## The Realities of Depression

"Every age yearns for a more beautiful world. The deeper the desperation and the depression about the confusing present, the more intense that yearning." **Johan Huizinga**

Depression is a mental disorder that affects not only the mind with its multiple moods, but also the overall wellness of the body as well as the whole being of an individual. Depression is an inner struggle striving to escape from the harsh realities of life.

## The Origin

"Depression begins with disappointment. When disappointment festers in our soul, it leads to discouragement." **Joyce Meyer**

Man is inherently desirous of *happiness*. We all want to become happy; without happiness, human existence may have become meaningless. Therefore, we all want to *avoid* unhappiness, and this self-defense mechanism may then develop into addictive habit patterns that have ultimately become some of the characteristics of our individual personality, affecting *how* we think. In other words, to avoid unhappiness, we may subconsciously begin to "lose contact with our realities" and thus become the persons we are not supposed to be. Depression is a mental struggle against unhappiness that an individual wishes to avoid, and in the process becomes a *different* person—a person with ever-changing moods and temperaments.

To illustrate, a baby or toddler—even well-fed, dry, and comfortable—may cry because he or she wants happiness, which is not being separated from the parents; crying or screaming is the only self-defense mechanism against being separated and feeling unhappy. As that baby or toddler continues to grow, that *normal* child will ultimately learn the reality that to be separated from the parents is just a normal and necessary part and parcel of life and maturity.

However, the mental and emotional growth and maturity of that same child may not be consistent with his or her physical growth and mental maturity, and this inconsistency or disparity may subsequently lead to many mental and emotional problems later in life, such as recklessly driving a car, engaging promiscuously in sex, taking drugs or addicting to alcohol. If the mental and emotional problems are not properly and fully addressed and resolved, that same adolescent turning into a young adult may continue to develop more problems, such as compulsive gambling or shopping sprees. As that same individual continues to grow and mature, there may be many other problems that crop up along his or her life journey, including problems in career, marriage, family, health, money, and among many others. All these life problems and challenges may continue to create more behavioral patterns, which are only the manifestations of that individual's desperate struggle against the unhappiness associated with emotional, mental, and physical problems; they are just the self-defense addictive behaviors of that individual striving desperately to overcome depression. In other words, that individual simply wants to *avoid* the un-happiness resulting from the many life problems and challenges encountered but unresolved.

## Unattainable Happiness

> "The greatest happiness is to know the source of unhappiness." **Fyodor Dostoevsky**

Depression is no more than a personal struggle against unattainable happiness, which is the essence of life and living. Therefore, almost everybody is always in quest of happiness. Sadly, to many, the quest for happiness is forever unreachable—just like a carrot-and-stick in front of a mule; the more pain inflicted on the mule by the stick: the more desire the mule demonstrates to reach out for the forever unattainable carrot in front. In many ways, a depressed individual is just like that mule with self-inflicted pain, which is the depression—the more unhappy that individual feels, the more depressed that individual will become, and the longer that vicious cycle of depression will continue, only plunging that depressed individual deeper into a fathomless black hole of despair and hopelessness. Depression is no more than a mental manifestation of the forever unattainable happiness that an individual strives to seek.

But why is human happiness so elusively and evasively unreachable and unattainable? The answer is, surprisingly, quite simple: happiness has to do with one's perceptions of life experiences, and thus the thinking mind plays a pivotal role in that respect. That is to say, human happiness and the human mind are inter-related; without profound human wisdom, the pursuit of happiness is like wandering in the wilderness without a compass and a road map. Indeed, true human wisdom holds the key to opening the door to understanding true human happiness.

Given the close connection between depression and happiness, understanding true human happiness may help a depressed individual overcome his or her depression.

## The Causes

> "You largely constructed your depression. It wasn't given to you. Therefore, you can deconstruct it." **Albert Ellis**

Although unhappiness is the underlying cause of depression, there are many other factors that may actually cause or trigger the onset of depression, because depression does not just happen by itself. If you have the attitude of "my way, or no way" and when you do not have the things you want "your way," you may then become more easily susceptible and vulnerable to depression.

## *Disappointment and frustration*

Disappointment and frustration are most common experiences, and they can be due to just about anything in life. But one of the most common sources is *people*: from one's spouse who does not meet one's expectations; from one's children, who are disobedient or rebellious to one's values and principles; from one's parents who do not approve of one's behavior and temperament, or, even worse, who wish they had never given birth to one.

Disappointment and frustration are more acutely felt when an individual has a distinct and strong ego-self, who loves himself or herself more than anyone else.

## Self-criticism and self-denial

Self-acceptance is an important element in the art of living well. We must all learn to accept ourselves as who we are, and not as who we wish we were. We must never cherish unrealistic expectations of ourselves, which may lead to low self-esteem. In other words, a perfectionist, ironically enough, may become more easily susceptible to the ultimate lack of self-esteem, which is often expressed in depression.

If you cannot accept yourself as who you are in spite of your imperfections and shortcomings, how can you accept others as who they are? If you do not love yourself as who you are, how can you love others as who they are? The bottom line: self-acceptance holds the key to having better relationships with others, which is frequently the source of human happiness.

## Comparison and contrast

There was an ancient Chinese fable of a stonecutter who worked so hard cutting stones that he often felt stressed and depressed.

One day, while standing behind a huge stone where he was cutting his stones, he looked up at the sky, and saw the beautiful sun. Then, he wished he were the sun that could give warmth and sunshine to everyone on earth. A fairy came to him and granted him his wish, so he became the sun.

For a while, he was happy and contented. Then, one day, a big cloud came over, blocked out everything from his view, and he could not see what was below. He became distressed and unhappy, and wished he were the cloud, instead of the sun. Again, the fairy came to his rescue, and granted him his wish. He became the cloud, and began drifting and floating happily and peacefully in the sky.

After a while, a strong wind came and scattered the cloud in different directions. Now, he wished he were the strong wind that could blow away anything and everything that stood in his way. Again, the fairy made his wish come true: he became the strong wind, blowing here and there. For a while, he was happy and contented.

Then, one day, he found out that he could not blow away the big stone behind which he used to cut stones. Worse, he was stuck there, going nowhere. Now, finally, he began to realize that was where he belonged. He made his one last wish to become the stonecutter that he used to be. The fairy granted him his last wish, and now he was contented to be the stonecutter again.

The moral of the fable: any comparison and contrast between self and others—or even between the current self and the self in the past—is often a stumbling block to self-contentment, the lack of which will direct one's thoughts inward and generate depression. Indeed, if you are discontent with what you have or what you are, while matching an area of your own deficiency with that of someone else's obvious strength, you are in fact preparing the groundwork for your own depression. It is just that simple!

## Despair and despondency

Feeling trapped in a dire situation or circumstance with no foreseeable exit only distresses the mind. It could be any situation or circumstance, such as getting an unwanted pregnancy, having several children early in a marriage saddled with many financial burdens but with no vocational skills, being stuck in a bad love relationship with no way out, and many other despairing and despondent situations.

## Adversity and loss

Adversity and loss are inevitable in life. Adversity may come in many different forms, such as accidents, injuries, and diseases; while loss can be physical loss, such as loss of mobility, material loss, such as loss of a home due to foreclosure, mental loss, such as loss of memory, spousal loss, such as separation or bereavement, and spiritual loss, such as loss of life purpose and meaningful existence in life.

## Inactivity and lack of goals

An inactive individual is more vulnerable to depression, because that individual spends most of his or her time drifting about and doing nothing in particular. By the same token, an individual lacking life goals ceases to struggle in life—that may explain why depression is more frequent among the senior and the elderly. Man is basically a goal-seeking creature. Therefore, after reaching one goal, an individual should set another higher goal in order to avoid the feeling of being letdown after the achievement of the goal, and thus setting off a depression.

The bottom line: never stay in a mental vacuum; always keep yourself mentally and physically busy and engaged, with something to look forward to. Remember, happy people always have strong goals, which have little to do with money, according to **Earl Nightingale**, an American author and motivational speaker.

## *Regret and self-pity*

A depressed individual often looks back at the past with anger and bitterness, accompanied by regret and self-pity. "What if" and "I wish it were" are always on the mind of that depressed individual, wishing things were different. Regret and self-pity always go hand-in-hand with that depressed individual.

## *Biological malfunction and chemical imbalance*

Of course, with the advancement of modern medicine, medical authorities have now attributed many cases of depression to biological malfunction, such as an abnormal thyroid, or imbalance of certain brain chemicals. However, it should be pointed out that it is difficult to determine whether it is the thinking mind or the chemical imbalance that actually causes the biological malfunctioning. The explanation is that an individual's own negative or self-destructive thinking patterns may also ultimately lead to the chemical and hormonal imbalance in that individual.

Therefore, we should always look at the whole picture, and not just a part of it; after all, depression is a complex and complicated disease of the mind, and we are also living in a world of depression.

## The Symptoms

"It's a recession when your neighbor loses his job; it's a depression when you lose yours."
**Harry S Truman**

Depression begins in the mind, affecting the emotions and feelings of an individual, with some of the most common symptoms, including the following:

## *Lethargy and loss of appetite*

A depressed individual begins to feel lethargy and listlessness without any apparent reason. The mind simply refuses to function, causing physical tiredness and even loss of appetite.

## *Involuntary tendency to weep*

Many depressed individuals get the sudden "weeps"—a tale-telling sign of the beginning of depression.

## *Irritability and hostility*

A depressed individual, who is often passive or inactive, may express irritability towards someone who wishes to activate that individual physically or mentally.

A depressed individual may also initially express hostility directed towards someone who has rejected or insulted him or her, before turning that hostility inward at himself or herself.

## *Sadness and hopelessness*

The most common symptom of depression, of course, is feeling sadness and hopelessness that may drag over a long period of time. The almost worldwide symptom of all depressed people is *withdrawal* from others, including the loved ones due to their loss of affection for self and others.

## Points to Remember

- We are all depressed, with no exception; just do not deny or stigmatize depression.
- We are living in a world of depression that can make us unhappy in many different ways, and we are all vulnerable.
- Depression is always an inner struggle against unhappiness and insecurity; it is a deliberate and desperate but futile attempt to lose contact with the realities of life. Depression is no more than a mental escape from the inescapable.

# TWO

## THE THINKING MIND

"It stands to the everlasting credit of science that by acting on the human mind it has overcome man's insecurity before himself and nature." **Albert Einstein**

Depression is all about the *mind*—the "thinking" mind; more specifically, *how* the mind functions. The human mind plays a pivotal role in depression: it could be the underlying "cause" of many problems related to depression; on the other hand, it could also be the "antidote" of depression. That is to say, the human mind is a double-edged sword: it could create many "problems" for depression, as well as provide many "solutions" to depression.

The thinking mind plays several major roles in your life, especially in relation to depression.

Life is about experiences, which are composed of *thoughts* of those experiences by the human mind. According to **James Allen**, the author of *As A Man Thinketh*, men are "makers of themselves" and the human mind is the "master-weaver, by both of the inner garment of character and the outer garment of circumstance." Accordingly, you may have become who you and what you are by way of your thinking mind over the years; in short, you are the sum of your own thoughts. Therefore, your thinking mind plays a pivotal role in your life.

First and foremost, you must fully understand the major roles of your mind in your everyday life and living, and *how* it may work for you or against you with respect to your depression.

## Perceptions and Realities

"Everything you perceive, externally, is the manifestation of some internal part of you. If it was not, it would not be present in your perceived reality." **Tony Warrick**

Your mind perceives all your life experiences through your five senses: seeing, hearing, touching, smelling, and tasting. To most people, seeing is the most important perception; however, what they *see* may not be the *absolute* reality, because their visual perceptions may be conditioned by what they see, and distorted by many other factors during the processing of their perceptions. Remember, it is the *intuition* of your soul that really perceives your reality. The wise have known for a long time that what we know through our eyes are not the same as the intuition of the soul. If that is the case, sadly, most people rely solely on what they see, thinking that "seeing is believing," and thus lose themselves in external things.

As an illustration, in 1997, **Richard Alexander** from Indiana was convicted as a serial rapist because one of the victims and her fiancé insisted that he was the perpetrator based on what they saw with their own eyes. However, the convicted man was exonerated and released in 2001 based on new DNA science and other forensic evidence. Experts explained that a traumatic emotional experience, such as a rape, could "distort" the perception of an individual.

The truth is that your brain is composed of grey matters

and neurons or nerve cells that transmit information and messages; they are the building blocks of your brain for the processing of all your perceptions. Neurons are responsible for all your behaviors in the form of perceptions, which trigger a mental process that results in an action or an emotion. If the process becomes instinctive or habitual, then the output in the form of an action or an emotion is also automatic and predictable. That is how *attitudes* and *habits* are formed, including the fight-or-flight response to any dangerous situation. This automatic or spontaneous mental processing is often not "by choice." The fact of the matter is that this "learned" mental processing is responsible for the way you think and act, for your beliefs and emotions, for you attitudes and prejudices, as well as for your decisions or indecisions—in other words, every aspect of your life experiences.

**Descartes**, the great French philosopher, made his famous statement: "I think, therefore I am." That means, you think, and your thoughts then become who and what you *think* you are. But that may not be the *real* you

In many ways, the human brain is like a computer program. Your whole being is like the computer hardware with the apparatus of a mind, a body, and the five senses. The lenses, through which you see yourself, others, and the whole world around you, are the software that has been continuously programmed by your thoughts, your past and present experiences, as well as your own expectations and those of others projected into the future. In other words, you and nobody else have programmed your own present mindset. All these years, you might have been trapped in a constricted sense of self that has prevented you from knowing and being who you really are. Your "conditioned" mindset might have erroneously made you "think" and "believe" that you are who and what you are right now; but nothing could be further from the truth.

## The Conscious and the Subconscious Mind

"Our thoughts are mainly controlled by our subconscious, which is largely formed before the age of 6, and you cannot change the subconscious mind by just thinking about it. That's why the power of positive thinking will not work for most people. The subconscious mind is like a tape player. Until you change the tape, it will not change." **Bruce Lipton**

We all have both a conscious and a subconscious mind. Simply put, your conscious mind does all the *active thinking*: selectively recording whatever data and information you want to remember and reserve them for future use, while discarding whatever you consciously think is irrelevant or inapplicable to you in the future. Your subconscious mind, on the other hand, absorbs *everything indiscriminately* that you are exposed to, and stores it at the back of your mind in the form of emotions, feelings, and memories.

Originally, your mind is like that of a baby, which is a blank sheet of paper. Your thinking begins with your five senses—*how* they perceive and interpret your own life experiences. Then all these emotional, mental, and physical sensations become your thoughts or memories stored at the back of your subconscious mind. So, whenever you experience a similar sensation, your conscious mind will automatically go back to your subconscious mind to look for more clues, relevant information, or guidelines, and send out different messages back to your conscious mind, instructing it to act or react accordingly. As an illustration, a baby, who previously experienced a pleasantly tickling sensation, will begin to giggle and laugh, feeling pleased, when being tickled again, as soon as the subconscious mind sends to the conscious mind the message of that pleasant sensation previously experienced.

Essentially, while your conscious mind is just about to make all your everyday life choices and decisions, your subconscious mind is, in fact, *controlling* and *directing* your conscious mind from behind the scene without letting you know; that is why it is called a "subconscious" mind.

Gradually and accumulatively, all your life experiences with their own respective messages—the pleasant as well as the unpleasant, the positive as well as the negative—are all stored at the back of your subconscious mind in the form of data and memories. Over the long haul, millions and billions of such experiences and messages have become the raw materials with which you subconsciously weave the fabrics of your life, making you *who* and *what* you have now become—or so you *think*. In other words, they have now become your so-called "realities."

But they are *not* your realities. The truth of the matter is that they are no more than your own thinking, controlled and dominated by your own subconscious mind. To illustrate, say, your conscious mind tells you to eat a healthful meal, but your subconscious mind—loaded with the images and messages of many TV commercials of mouth-watering junk food, as well as your own past delectable experiences of some of them—may tell you something totally different, and you may end up eating a burger and French fries.

## The Personality Creation

"The 'self-image' is the key to human

personality and human behavior. Change the self image and you change the personality and the behavior." **Maxwell Maltz**

Your "thinking" mind is responsible for creating not only your so-called "realities" based on your perceptions of your life experiences, but also your personality, which also plays a pivotal role in your living in a world of depression.

It is your human nature to identify yourself with your thoughts created by your own thinking mind. This identity begins to relate to more thoughts, both past and present, as well as their projections into the future as desires and expectations. These accumulative thoughts begin to take shape and form your ego-self, which *all* of us have, because it is the identity that separates and distinguishes us from others.

But is that ego-self for real? Or what exactly is the ego-self?

Simply look at yourself in front of a mirror. What do you see? A *self* reflection. Is it for real? Can you touch it? Not really; it is only a *reflection* of someone real—the real *you* in front of the mirror!

Your ego-self is your *self-perceived* personality. Just like the reflection in the mirror, it is not the *real* you.

Now, do something slightly different. Place a baby—if there is one immediately available—in front of the mirror. Now. see what happens. The baby may crawl towards the baby in the mirror. Why? It is because the baby in front of the mirror thinks that the baby in the mirror is *another* baby, and not his or her own reflection.

Likewise, your ego-self may look real to you, but it is *not* real It is only a *reflection* of your own thoughts; that is, your ego self is what you think or even wish you were. The ego-self is formed over the years, transforming you into someone else that you are not. Your only one true life obligation is to be the person standing in front of the mirror, and not the *reflection* of that person in the mirror.

Your ego-self, which is formed by your thoughts, often become your attachments. Too many attachments to your ego-self may become problematic, leading to depression.

## The Unhappy Personality

There are those who are forever unhappy due to an unhappy childhood, an unfulfilled adult life, and many unhappy life experiences throughout their life journeys. They have made indelible imprints on their minds, making them see only the problems, instead of the potentials ahead of them. They do not want to live, but they just do not die. Not wanting or knowing how to purposely end their lives, they just drift on, or simply live a reckless life in hope of an early demise.

They have suffered and gone through too much in their lives. They do not know how to cope with their life problems and how to deal with their life challenges. They have despaired and become helpless, and depression is their only escape from the realities they strive to avoid. They are forever the unhappy ones because unhappiness has become their brain chemicals.

## The Neither-Happy-Nor-Unhappy Personality

There are those who have always been only spectators, instead of participants, of life; they are forever sitting on the sidelines of life, observing others and never thinking that they could be a part of it. They always believe that life is not worth taking chances because their minds have been filled with many assumptions that they are not competent enough to get involved. Inactivity and passivity play a major role in their lives. They may not like their current situations, but they do not know how and where to start to change them. Even if they have the know-how, they do not want to do it, or unless someone else would do it for them. Life is too much for them; they just stay back and stay put, not taking any chance or exerting any effort, while they try to get by with whatever they have. They never see the need to take the initiative to create a better life for themselves.

If they just do not die, they just carry on with their lives with different episodes of high and low, always wondering why they do not have what they wish they had, or why others are always having what they are not having.

## The To-Be-Happy Personality

There are those who are always in quest of happiness. They have the problematic mindset of "better" and "more" in their endless quest for careers, relationships, and material comforts that have become the sole objectives of their personal happiness. Their to-be-happiness just keeps them always wanting "better" and "more" in order to feel happy or happier.

## The Happy Personality

There are those who have the wisdom to understand that true happiness requires both action and effort, that happiness is only a moment-to-moment feeling, and that happiness never lasts.

Indeed, happiness is *feeling good* about oneself, and it requires one to take some actions in order to feel good about oneself. It should be pointed out that elated feelings, such as happiness, satisfaction, and fulfillment, are not the natural and normal resting states of the human mind; therefore, one must take a *deliberate* action in order to achieve and activate those innate mental states. The only explanation is that our ancestors in the Stone Age did not naturally or instinctively feel comfortable, secure, and satisfied with their status quo. They certainly did not pass those genes on to us. They had to fight to survive; by the same token, we all must make a *conscious* effort to take some actions in order to feel good, happy, and satisfied.

Remember, true human happiness is a process, a way of living, involving some actions to change the consciousness of thinking. It is no more than the ability to experience joy when good things happen; the ability to feel satisfaction when goals are achieved; the ability to cope with problems, the ability to adapt to changes, and the ability to give meaning and purpose to life.

## The conclusion

In general, the above four different happiness mindsets are responsible for the creation of different personalities. Not only the characteristics of one type of mindset may overlap those of another, but also one type of mindset may become another; it is all in the consciousness of an individual's thinking mind.

### The Thinking Mind and Human Happiness

"If we could get your subconscious mind to agree with your conscious mind about being happy, that's when your positive thoughts work." **Bruce Lipton**

Given that happiness has a direct link to depression, it is

therefore important to understand *how* the thinking mind may affect the mental state of happiness.

Generally speaking, the purpose of life and living is two-fold: to *enjoy* life, and to *expand* happiness.

But how can one enjoy life if one is not happy by nature, or how can one expand happiness if one has no idea what happiness is all about? Therefore, it is critically important to *understand* how the thinking mind works, and how it can make you happy or unhappy over the long haul.

## The Happiness Myths

Happiness is only an abstraction, a far-fetched thought that is often elusive and evasive; it is difficult not only to define but also to understand. To further the complication, happiness often creates certain misleading myths.

### *The myth: the happiness sources*

It is always a myth that *abundant wealth*, *good health*, and *satisfying relationships*—what most people crave and pursue in their lives—will bring them happiness. Abundant wealth, good health, and satisfying relationships are only the *byproducts* of happiness; they do not cause or bring true and lasting happiness in real life.

To illustrate, many lottery winners attest to their experiences of temporary ecstatic happiness, and nearly all winners confess that their winning has ultimately made them miserable and unhappy for various reasons. Maybe once the initial stimulus of sudden wealth and the drastic changes of lifestyle have worn off, they ultimately return to their original baseline level of happiness or unhappiness. Or, maybe, according to some experts, having too much pleasure—what is known as "eustress"—could also cause stress, just as lacking in pleasure might be stressful to the many have-nots.

## The myth: the happiness effort

It is also a myth that happiness is something that can be pursued with willpower and effort. The Bible rightly says that pursuing happiness is just "like chasing the wind." (**Ecclesiastes** 2:11)

Effort does not necessarily bring happiness; it only creates the *illusion* of an environment that is conducive to temporary happiness. To illustrate, one may work diligently in one's career to excel and to get to the very top of the profession only to find that one has a terminal illness, or has incurred a debilitating accident. For example, **Steve Job**, the co-founder of Apple computers, had his life cut short by pancreatic cancer at the height of his successful business career.

Pursuing happiness may be only a fantasy fueled by temporary moments of happiness, because aging, illnesses, misfortunes, and ultimately death plague all alike; in other words, *impermanence* cuts short all human efforts and endeavors to bring happiness. We are all aware of the fact that impermanence is an ultimate leveler of everybody and everything, but many of us still choose to delude ourselves into thinking otherwise. Denial only fosters the myth that if there is a will then there must be a way to attaining happiness, and that all it requires is the human effort to make any dream come true.

## The Attributes of True Happiness

Advertising, consumerism, and the media have all mesmerized us into believing that happiness is one of the basic human rights that we are all entitled to. The truth of the matter is that true happiness is, surprisingly, *simple* and *effortless*, because it comes from within, and not from without; it is part of self, and is natural to human life and existence. It is all in the mind—that is, *how* we think.

If that is the case, then why is that some people are happy, while others are unhappy?

There is so much truth in what **Leo Tolstoy**, the famous Russian author, said in very beginning of his celebrated novel *Anna Karenina*: "Happy families are alike, and unhappy families are unhappy in their own way." So, those who are happy and those who are unhappy must have shared some common attributes or characteristics that predispose them to happiness or unhappiness.

## The unhappy people

The unhappy people may have the following common characteristics:

### Identity crisis

They do not know *who* they really are. That is, they may have falsely identified themselves with something in the world they are living in, such as "I am a successful businessman" or "I am a good mother."

Once they have created for themselves their false identities, they naturally feel the need to protect and preserve their self-created images. In doing so, they desperately want to *control* and *protect* their destinies, such as avoiding what they fear might taint their preserved identities, or repeating what they previously did in order to sustain and substantiate their identities.

As an example, a "successful businessman" might want

to overwork in order to avoid in future all possible failures in his or her business, or to repeat in future all his or her past successful business endeavors.

As another example, a "good mother" might strive to control the behaviors of her children in order to control and shape them into the individuals she wants them to become to prove that she is indeed a "good mother."

In the process of protecting and sustaining that identity, stress is not only unduly created but also aggravated by all outcomes falling short of the individual's expectations. Nowadays, many people are living just to escape their yesterday's pains and to anticipate their tomorrow's pleasures; unfortunately, they are on the road to more unhappiness, and not less.

The bottom line: you are who you are, and *not* who you would like to become.

## Not letting go

The unhappy people simply refuse to let go of what they think belong *permanently* to them; they anticipate what they think they rightly deserve through their efforts to control or influence the outcomes of events in their lives. They are afraid of any unforeseeable change, especially death that puts an end to everything they have delusively created for themselves.

## *The happy people*

The happy people are wise because they know not only how to *live* but also how to *survive* in a world of depression.

## Knowing the ultimate truths

The truly happy people are those who understand that the only permanent cure for unhappiness is *enlightenment*, which is the profound human wisdom to know who they are, and what life is all about. True happiness lies within the true self; it comes from knowing the ultimate truths about everything in life.

## Living a simple life

In addition, the happy people always live a simple life, which is the essence of life and living. They have little or no attachment because they understand that everything is impermanent and subject to change and demise. Therefore, craving for more may also imply getting more problems when things do not last.

Remember, you have to be always *conscious* of your thinking mind in order to better *understand* your perceptions and then *change* them so that they may become a glass half-full, and not a glass half-empty.

## **Points to Remember**

- It is the thinking mind that can get one into or out of depression.
- The human mind perceives all life experiences, and perceptions create the so-called "realities" that may not be real, except in the mind.
- The "perceived realities" determine the happy or unhappy mindset of an individual.
- Consciousness is the pathway to understanding the need to *change* perceptions to change the realities.

# THREE

## THE HUMAN WISDOM

"It is the mark of an educated mind to be able to entertain a thought without accepting it."
**Aristotle**

Given that realities are created by perceptions that come from the thinking mind, you must change *how* your mind thinks in order to change your perceptions to change the "perceived realities" that are responsible for depression.

Depression is a problematic disorder of the thinking mind, causing multi-faceted problems to an individual living in the physical word. The only solutions to these problems must also come from the same source, that is, the thinking mind that has created those problems in the first place. Solving all these problems with medications is not the ultimate solution. Initially they may suppress the symptoms of depression for a while, but they do not permanently eliminate the underlying problems. Using anti-depression medications to uplift the mood of a depressed individual is like giving a different drug to an addict, or an extra dose of alcohol to an alcoholic. In addition, most anti-depressants have many undesirable side effects, and one of which is weight gain that may become another weight management problem, and thus triggering another depression.

Given that depression originates from the thinking

mind, the antidote of depression must also come from the very same source, that is, the thinking mind. To effectively and efficiently deal with the thinking mind, human wisdom is indispensable.

## Wisdom and Knowledge

"Any fool can know. The point is to understand." **Albert Einstein**

Wisdom is not the same as knowledge in that the former has much to do with the processing of data and information by the thinking mind, while the latter has much to do with the acquisition of facts and information by the thinking mind. Wisdom is the clarity of the thinking mind to see things as they really are, and not as what they are supposed to be; knowledge, on the other hand, is the capability of the thinking mind to use the information collected to solve all the daily problems encountered. Being knowledgeable may imply only smartness, but it does not necessarily suggest wisdom. After all, humans are all limited in their capacity and capability to acquire knowledge, which is itself unlimited. Therefore, to use what is limited for the unlimited is irrational. Wisdom, on the other hand, is to use mind power, which is potentially unlimited, to apply the limited knowledge acquired to understand the true nature of self, others, and the things around.

## The Wisdom to Be Self-Conscious

"The key to growth is the introduction of higher dimensions of consciousness into our awareness." **Lao Tzu**

Consciousness is *everything*; if you are not conscious, you are not living your life, if not already dead.

What is consciousness? Being conscious is a "special quality of the mind" that permits us to *know* both that we exist and that the things around us *also* exist. Surprisingly, many of us may not have this consciousness.

Life is an inner journey that often requires consciousness of the body and the mind, together with that of the soul or spirit, to continue making its progress in the right direction in order to reach its final destination. Sadly, since the beginning of time, many people have traveled on the same journey of life but without reaching their desired destinations because they simply lack their consciousness of the body and the mind, not to mention that of the soul or spirit, to guide them along that long and winding life journey with its many detours and sidetracks.

Consciousness comes from the mind, which is created by the brain. **Hippocrates** (460 - 370 BC), the father of modern medicine, was one of the first scientists to observe and notice that people with brain damage tended to lose their mental abilities. He realized that the mind is created by the brain, and that the mind crumbles piece by piece as the brain dies.

The human brain creates the consciousness of the mind, and thus giving all humans their pleasures and displeasures, happiness and unhappiness, as well as other positive and negative feelings and emotions. These human perceptions then become their experiences which are stored in their minds as memories generating their subsequent thoughts—together they then become the byproducts with which they weave the realities in their lives.

Consciousness is the capability of your thinking mind to see *how* and *why* certain perceptions occur and affect your thinking mind. Without this consciousness, which is knowing what is happening in the mind, you just obediently follow what your mind tells you to do. That is to say, you have become a slave to your thinking mind, instead of being the master of your own thoughts.

Are you conscious of your mind, or what your mind is thinking right now?

You may be conscious of your thinking mind *if* you are also conscious of your breathing. Life is made up of many breaths. For thousands of years, the Chinese have believed that the lifespan of an individual is determined by the number of breaths assigned to that individual at birth. That explains why traditional Chinese exercises, such as *Qi Gong* and *Tai Chi*, focus so much on the art of breathing, especially on extending the breaths, which holds the key to longevity. Western science has already attested to the fact that tortoise, with the longest lifespan in the animal kingdom, has also the longest breath, while rodent, with the shortest lifespan, has the shortest breath. Therefore, the consciousness of your breaths is a reflection of your own consciousness of life, as well as of many other things in your life.

Consciousness of breaths begins with breathing. Are you constantly conscious of your breaths—your breathing in and breathing out? Most people are not. Breathing is the most subconscious and yet the most important moment-to-moment activity in human life. Unfortunately, many of us are not conscious of our breathing; we just take it for granted. The Bible has made references to the importance of the breath from God, which is not only life itself but also *divine understanding*.

And the LORD God formed man *of* the dust
of the ground, and breathed into his nostrils

the breath of life; and man became a living being. (**Genesis** 2:7)

But *there is* a spirit in man, And the breath of the Almighty gives him understanding. (**Job** 32:8)

Consciousness of breaths also suggests consciousness of self. Self-consciousness is, in fact, *everything* in your life and living. Self-consciousness is your mental awareness of self, others, and the world around you. Self-consciousness is mindfulness of what is happening to you and around you. Without this consciousness of the mind, you are not living; you are simply existing, making yourself become more vulnerable to depression.

## The Wisdom to Ask Questions

"The art and science of asking questions is the source of all knowledge." **Thomas Berger**

"Judge a man by his questions rather than his answers." **Voltaire**

Asking questions and seeking answers is deep thinking, which is the only pathway to attaining human wisdom. **Albert Einstein** once said, "Thinking is difficult; that's why so few people do it."

Thinking is a process of self-intuition through asking relevant questions in order to create self-consciousness and self-introspection. It is the natural habit of the human mind to try to solve problems by asking questions. Through solving problems, the mind can then make things *happen*. Asking relevant questions is self-empowerment of the human mind to create wisdom because it creates the intent of the mind to learn, to discover, and then to *change* the mind to change the self. Change is one of the most difficult human endeavors. There is a Chinese saying: "It is easier to change the landscape than to change the human character." Without that change, however, it is often difficult to adapt to the many life changes occurring along the life journey. Life without any change becomes static, boring, and ultimately meaningless and unhappy.

Asking questions and then seeking answers through the conscious mind may be the pathway to self-enlightenment. After all, throughout one's life journey, one has to ask many different questions at different stages, and seeking different answers from the questions asked. In order to reach the final destination of one's life journey, the wisdom in asking the right questions and seeking appropriate answers is a necessity, and not an option.

When you ask self-intuitive questions, you begin to empower your mind to seek self-enlightening answers to the questions asked. This internal mental consciousness is just the beginning of true human wisdom. The answer to every question you ask may change over time because life is forever changing, and changes are self-transformative. The more questions you ask, the clearer your mind becomes, and the more ready and receptive you are to receive the answers. That is *how* you enhance and increase your wisdom by asking questions and seeking answers.

Although asking questions is a self-learning process, do not seek absolute answers from the questions asked; more importantly, do not seek answers that sometimes cannot be given to you. The most important thing in questions-and-answers is to *experience* everything in the process, not just to pursue knowledge. As a matter of fact, knowledge can help, but it can also hinder. When you only follow what you *know*, and forget what you *feel*, you can easily be led down the wrong pathway. Remember, extensive knowledge and logical reasoning may not necessarily compound human wisdom.

Live every question you are going to ask yourself, and live in its presence. Be patient towards all those questions that you may not have an answer right away. True enlightenment may dawn on you one day when you find yourself asking no more questions because you already have all the answers; *that* is the ultimate self-enlightenment, which is the essence of profound human wisdom.

## The Wisdom to Look Inside

"You can only get outside yourself by looking inside" **Tonya Hurley**

"Your vision will become clear only when you can look into your own heart. Who looks outside, dreams; who looks inside, awakes." **Carl Jung**

"A beggar has been sitting by the side of a road for over thirty years. One day a stranger walked by. 'Spare some change?' mumbled the beggar, mechanically holding out his old baseball cap. 'I have nothing to give you,' said the stranger. Then he asked: 'What's that you are sitting on?' 'Nothing,' replied the beggar. 'Just an old box. I have been sitting on it for as long as I can remember.' 'Ever looked inside?' asked the stranger. 'No,' said the beggar. 'What's the point? There's nothing in there.' 'Have a look inside,' insisted the stranger. The beggar managed to prey open the lid. With astonishment, disbelief, and elation, he saw that the box was filled with gold."

The story above is taken from the beginning of the book *The Power of Now* by **Eckhart Tolle**.

Look inside! True human wisdom is already *inside* you, but you just have to *look*!

Yes, *looking inside* holds the key to understanding and attaining true human wisdom, which comes from within and not from without. Life is a journey of self-discovery, but it is *your* journey, and not someone else's. Therefore, you must look inside *you* to discover your true self, what you need and not what you want, as well as the ultimate truths of all things that happen to you and around you.

Looking inside requires consciousness of the being that is deep within you.

## The Wisdom to Understand

"Knowing yourself is the beginning of all wisdom." **Aristotle**

"Everything that irritates us about others can lead us to an understanding of ourselves." **Carl Jung**

"All truths are easy to understand once they are discovered; the point is to discover them." **Galileo Galilei**

## Assumptions and Attitudes

The human mind is intelligent in that it inherently knows how to organize life experiences into different patterns so that they may be easily and readily available. These thinking patterns are just like a filing cabinet with its many different drawers and many different folders, each with a different tag to indicate what that is. That filing cabinet has become the subconscious of the individual who has created it; whenever looking for any information, that individual would automatically go and search through the many drawers and folders in his or her filing cabinet.

We all have our own individual *automatic* thinking patterns to help us organize our thoughts, just like looking through our own filing cabinets, and thus enabling us to make our own subjective observations, generalizations, predictions, and even our expectations. Automatically, they might have become the many *implicit assumptions* to help us see how life works for or against us.

Indeed, we are living in an assumptive world with just too many implicit assumptions that, ironically enough, may often become stumbling blocks in our lives—in particular, in *how* we think. Being conscious of the subconscious may help us see the ultimate truths in all our own implicit assumptions—the truths that nothing is set in stone, and that we can still teach an old dog new tricks. The truth of the matter is that we have to *rethink* our minds in order to believe that there are too many *exceptions* to all our implicit assumptions that are derived from our own observations, often leading to our generalizations and expectations that we might have subconsciously created for ourselves. Our consciousness of the subconscious may help us live the rest of our lives very *differently*, and not as what we might have erroneously assumed.

Always use your consciousness to look deeply into what is *really* happening in your thinking mind—or *how* it might have got in your own way by providing you with only the superficial observations leading to your over-generalizations that are often followed by your own automatic predictions and expectations in the implicit assumptive world. Let your consciousness deliver you from the half-truths and untruths you might have been floundering in all these years that have become the underlying causes of your depression.

As an illustration, your daughter is about to get married; she plans to have a family soon; she is looking for a house to buy—the fact that she will be "happily married" is based on your automatic thinking pattern of implicit assumptions. But the reality is that there might be many exceptions to all your assumptions: the marriage might be canceled at the last moment; the pregnancy might be unsuccessful; the new home might be destroyed in a wildfire, a hurricane, or a tornado; and so on and so forth.

Life is full of changes, and many of which are sudden and unpredictable—they often become the exceptions to your implicit assumptions. With consciousness of thinking, you may even find more exceptions to all your automatic assumptions; with more exceptions, you may then become not only less resistant but also more adaptable to all the unpredictable changes encountered and experienced along your life journey. Do not let your automatic assumptions limit what you will be able to see and experience in life. If you just continue to live, the sky is the limit.

Always challenge and change your assumptions; they are no more than your selective attention to what you want to believe. Over the years, have you been looking for jobs that do not challenge your expectations? Do you always select your favorite TV news channels based on your assumptive preferences and expectations?

Maybe, now is the time to do what you normally do not do—or what is known as *reverse thinking.*

## Processing and Personality

We all process our experiences in different ways in

different phases of our lives. All our thoughts associated with all these experiences are indelibly etched in our subconscious minds, and inevitably creating our individual different feelings and emotions, both positive and negative ones, in different phases in our lives.

## *The development phase*

Throughout the early phase of growth and development, young children are exposed through their five senses to the world around them. Their minds begin to process whatever they perceive, generalize, and then apply them whenever and wherever they think appropriate—they have become the foundations of their own experiences and perceptions, which subsequently create the expectations in their adult lives. For example, if properly taught, they begin to show appreciation, as demonstrated by their saying their first "thank you."

During this critical first phase, their mental input is automatic and passive because their immature minds are unable to filter their mental input; their thoughts are merely a micro reflection of the minds of their parents. As they grow up, however, they may begin to learn how to "refuse" processing any unpleasant experience, or "interpret" it in the way they choose according to its relevance to their lives. Their selectivity then begins to alter how they process their life experiences in the future.

In this learning phase, children and young adults are learning incessantly, trying to understand and make sense out of the complex world they are living in. In this intensive learning phase, they begin to discern their respective roles they are going to play in the world they are living in, always looking for inspiration and direction from people around them, and not necessarily from their own parents.

## The transitional phase

Even though every phase of a person's life is important, none is more critical than the transitional phase from adolescence to adulthood. As young adults, the world around them becomes more complex and complicated. In addition, everything around them becomes increasingly exciting as experienced by the five senses, such as music and sex. But their self-delusions created by the way they process their experiences may also make them see more of the excitement and less of the reality of their world. This is a critical phase for most of them because it defines not only who they are but also what they value; it sets the foundation for the way that the rest of their lives is likely to turn out because their thoughts are a preview of what their future lives would be like.

## The consolidation phase

As they turn into full-grown adults, they begin to think more than just about themselves: they begin to focus more on the people around them. They may have their own life callings: career, health, love, or family; in other words, what they are meant to do with their lives. With passion and bliss, they may begin to define who they are. Being strong physically and mentally, they are in the most productive phase in their lives. During this phase, they merely respond and react, either positively or negatively, to the experiences presented to them in the form of career, marriage, and parenting.

This is a phase in which they consolidate their past experiences, and continue to build their future lives on that foundation. If they avail themselves of the opportunity to accept others as they are, and to become appreciative of what life has to offer, they will then develop the quality of acceptance in the form of love, compassion, and even forgiveness, which will have lasting effects on their future life experiences.

## *The letting go phase*

With advancement in age, and as age begins to take its toll on the body and the mind, most of the life habits that control how they should live have become well established. Their thoughts, based on decades of past experiences, now dominate their thinking mind, and hence control how they live the rest of their lives. At this point in time, it is difficult, if not impossible, to alter the way they process their experiences and perceptions, just as the saying goes: "It is difficult to teach an old dog new tricks."

In this final phase in their lives, unfortunately, they have to learn to let go of everything, whether they like it or not. Everything begins to slip from their lives: their youth, their health, and inevitably their minds too.

## Understanding Self

Now, look back at all the phases you have gone through so far, and try to recall *how* your mind had processed some of your perceptions of those past experiences in different phases of your life. More importantly, see if you now *understand* how your mind processing has defined the type of person you have now become. All the past happenings in your life were real to you, but the ways you *processed* and *perceived* them might have either positively or negatively affected your life over the past years. Because they have been stored in your subconscious mind, they might have given you valuable life lessons, or created delusions and self-deceptions that might not only confuse you but also lead you astray, making you depressed.

Now, you may have become aware that wisdom plays a pivotal role in *how* the mind processes life experiences and expectations.

## The Wisdom to Align and Balance

"In reaching for balance, we find alignment."
**Sue Krebs**

"The things bring you the greatest joy are in alignment with your purpose." **Jack Canfield**

Humans are given a physical body, a mind, and a soul or spirit. The body lives in the physical world, and is equipped with the five senses to live and survive in the physical environment. The mind, as the mediator between the body and the soul, is given the gift of free will, which is the freedom to process any input in the form of thoughts and sensations from both the body and the soul. That is to say, whenever we wish to do something, the soul intuitively provides the instinctive advice and judgment, the mind then carries out its analysis and interpretation, and the body eventually takes the appropriate action or decision of the mind. In other words, what we want to do and how we are going to do it are all within the control and power of the mind, which receives intuitively instructions from the soul, but makes the final decision to accept, reject, or modify the instructions.

Therefore, it is important that the body, the mind, and the soul are in balance and alignment with one another to attain the profound wisdom to understand the ultimate truths of all things, including the true self, which is self-enlightenment.

## Self-Enlightenment

Once your mind becomes enlightened, it will never go back to darkness again. But self-enlightenment is not easy to come by; it may require profound and unconventional human wisdom, such as that of **Lao Tzu**, also known as TAO wisdom.

## Points to Remember

- Depression originates from the thinking mind; therefore, overcome depression with the thinking mind.
- Wisdom is using unlimited mind power to apply limited human knowledge to understand self, others, and the things happening around in order to know the *hows* and the *whys* of depression.
- Wisdom is derived from asking questions and seeking answers to activate the thinking mind.
- Consciousness is looking inside self to find true wisdom, which always comes from within, and not from without.
- "Perceived" realities may not be the "real" realities due to distorted perceptions by the thinking mind, resulting in many implicit assumptions that form human attitudes and beliefs. Focus the mind on the many exceptions to all your implicit assumptions.
- Looking back at the different phases of personality development may shed some light on why you have

become the who and the what you are right now. Personality is manifested in the thinking mind.

- True human wisdom comes from the alignment of the body, the mind, and the soul—which is self-enlightenment.

# FOUR

## TAO WISDOM

### What Is TAO Wisdom?

TAO (道), also known as The Way or TAO wisdom, is the ancient wisdom from China more than two thousand six hundred years ago. It originated from the ancient classic *Tao Te Ching* (道德經), the only book written by **Lao Tzu** (老子) the Chinese sage, who was born with white hair—often considered a sign of old age and wisdom.

*Tao Te Ching* is an ancient Chinese classic on human wisdom. This unique piece of literature is one of the most translated books in human history. The book is a collection of Chinese wisdom poetry, in which the author expresses his wisdom in living life in all of its beauty and joy, as well as in all of its pain and sorrow. The language is simple and poetic, but controversial and paradoxical.

> "My words are easy to understand
> and easy to perform,
> Yet no man under heaven
> knows them or practices them."
> (Lao Tzu, *Tao Te Ching*, Chapter 70)

The word "TAO" describes what is indescribable, puts into words what is wordless, and gives sound to what is silent.

There are altogether 81 short chapters, expressed in only 5,000 words. It must be pointed out that there was no punctuation in the original text. Given that each word in the Chinese language may be capable of having multiple meanings, the text without any punctuation is open to many different interpretations. A plausible explanation is that Lao Tzu was very much reluctant to express his wisdom in words; after all, he believed that true human wisdom was wordless. As a matter of fact, according to the legend, at that time he was at the point of leaving China for Tibet when he was stopped at the city gate and was told by the guard that he had to put down his wisdom in words before he could leave the country. Deliberately and defiantly, he put down his wisdom concisely and precisely in only 5,000 words with no punctuation at all.

TAO wisdom is inspiring and intriguing. It is inspiring because Lao Tzu's wisdom is eternal and unconventional; it is intriguing because the wisdom is simple and open to different interpretations—just like the three blind men, touching different parts of an elephant, who try to describe what an elephant may look like.

To illustrate, the following is taken from the first chapter of *Tao Te Ching* with only 59 Chinese characters:

道可道，非常道。名可名，非常名。

無名天地之始;有名萬物之母。

故常無，欲以觀其妙;常有，欲以觀其徼
。

此兩者，同出而異名，同謂之玄。

玄之又玄，眾妙之門。

(the original Chinese text; the punctuation marks were subsequently added by scholars)

"The name that can be named is not the eternal name.
As nameless, it is the origin of all things; as named, it is the mother of 10,000 things.
Ever desireless, one can see the mystery of all things.
Ever desiring, one can see only their manifestations.
And the mystery itself is the doorway to all understanding."
(Lao Tzu, *Tao Te Ching*, Chapter 1)

The above is a very close, almost word-for-word, translation of the original Chinese text.

The following is my own translation in plain English, as well as my own interpretation, of the first chapter of *Tao Te Ching* (my own interpretation is given in brackets):

If we could understand the Creator or explain His ways, then He is no longer infinite and eternal. (Human wisdom is limited and therefore we can never completely understand the ways of Nature or the Creator.)
Mankind, once given a name with an identity, is only the source, but not the creator, of all things. (Man invents but does not create something out of nothing; only the Creator, who is nameless with no identity, creates everything out of nothing.)
Ever humble, we see the mystery of all things in the Creator's realm of creation. (With humility, we may understand why certain things were created.)
Ever boastful, we see only the manifestations

of all things created. (With pride, we see the wonders of our own inventions, but not the mystery of the Creator's creations.)

And the mystery itself is the pathway to attaining greater spirituality and further understanding of the Creator. (Not knowing everything leads to further understanding of the purpose of creation by the Creator.)

TAO wisdom is profound human wisdom that requires self-intuition to have greater understanding of the Creator, who is in control of everything created by Him; this further understanding may be instrumental in enhancing human wisdom. For this reason, paradoxically, TAO was later on evolved into a religion, known as Taoism (道教)), in China. However, it must be pointed out that TAO was never intended to be a religion or some religious belief by Lao Tzu; it was meant to show only what *true* human wisdom really is, and how to live according to that wisdom.

## The Essentials of TAO

## (1) An Empty Mind

TAO wisdom begins with having an empty mind. What is an empty mind? An empty mind is more than just "thinking out of the box": it is *reverse* thinking, that is, creating your own box of thinking. An empty mindset originated from Lao Tzu:

> "An empty mind with no craving and no expectation helps us let go.
> Being in the world and not of the world, we attain heavenly grace.

With heavenly grace, we become pure and
selfless.
And everything settles into its own perfect
place."
(Lao Tzu, *Tao Te Ching*, Chapter 3)

There was the story of a professor visiting a Zen master
to find out more about Zen, which is an Eastern
philosophy originated from TAO. In the beginning of the
visit, the professor kept on talking while the Zen master
served him tea. At some point, the Zen master kept
pouring tea into the teacup held by the professor even
though it was already brimming over. The moral of the
story is that one must have an empty mind *first* before one
can accept any new and unconventional idea. Likewise, to
intuit true human wisdom, one must have an empty mind
capable of reverse thinking.

An empty mindset frees us from the many shackles of
life that may have enslaved us, keeping us in bondage
without our knowing it. Are you the master or just a slave
of your own life? You are the master only when you have
complete control over your own mind, which controls how
well you live your life.

How do you gain control over your life in terms of your
career, human relationships, time management, daily stress,
and among many others? It is not easy because most of us
have a pre-conditioned mindset that we must do this and
do that in order to get what we want, or to be successful.

The bottom line: have an empty mind because there is
no formula for success; do not let your life careen out of
control by following what conventional wisdom says.

Just follow your heart, and not what others do or say.
Be yourself!

## (2) Simplicity in Living

TAO suggests simplicity in living. Life is complex, and contemporary living is complicated with its many emotional and material clutters and attachments. To live well, you must have TAO wisdom to live a simple life, letting go of all the trimmings of contemporary living. The desire for simplicity in living may accelerate the process of letting go as life progresses, giving you clarity of thinking, which is the only pathway to human wisdom.

> "Simplicity is clarity.
> It is a blessing to learn from those
> with humble simplicity.
>
> Those with an empty mind
> will learn to find the Way.
>
> The Way reveals the secrets of the universe:
> the mysteries of the realm of creation;
> the manifestations of all things created.
> The essence of the Way is to show us
> how to live in fullness and return to our
> origin."
> (Lao Tzu, *Tao Te Ching*, Chapter 65)

## (3) Mindfulness

To create an empty mind with clarity of thinking, you need mindfulness, which is acute mental awareness of self and others, as well as of your needs and not your wants.

Mindfulness is mental sharpness to know what is happening in the mind that brings about clarity of thinking, which is essential to human wisdom.

There is a close connection between the body and the mind. This body-mind connection in humans affects both the physical and the mental health of an individual, especially how that individual thinks, acts, and reacts. It is important to put the mind where the body is. Mindfulness begins with the body. Becoming mindful of your body in the present moment is putting your mind where your body is. This produces deep relaxation of both the body and mind—an essential element for clarity of thinking that is the only pathway to attaining true human wisdom.

> "watchful, like a man crossing a winter stream;
> alert, like a man aware of danger;
> courteous, like a visiting guest;
> yielding, like ice about to melt;
> simple, like a piece of uncarved wood;
> hollow, like a cave;
> opaque, like muddy water."
> (Lao Tzu, *Tao Te Ching*, Chapter 15)

> "To end our suffering,
> find our true nature.
>
> Stilling our thoughts,
> our needs become few.
> Following our thoughts,
> our distractions become more,
> and thus living in chaos.
>
> Enlightenment is our true nature.
> Meditation helps us find the origin,
> and thus ending our suffering."
> (Lao Tzu, *Tao Te Ching*, Chapter 52)

## (4) Living in the Present

According to Lao Tzu, only the present is real: the past was gone, and the future is uncertain and unpredictable. In the present moment, with clarity of mind, you may see the ultimate truths of self, others, and everything happening to you and around you. More importantly, you may even see your own past follies in identifying yourself with your thoughts that might have created your present ego-self.

Living in the present is an awakening to the realities of all things. It affords you an opportunity to look more *deeply* and *objectively* at any given event, allowing your mind to think more clearly, and thus separating the truths from the self-deceptions that might have been created in your own subconscious mind all along.

"Living in the present moment,
we find natural contentment.
We do not seek a faster lifestyle,
or a better place to be.
We need the essentials of life,
not its extra trimmings.

Living in the present moment,
we focus on the experience of the moment.
Thus, we enjoy every aspect of simple living,
and find contentment in everyone and in everything.

Living in contentment,
we grow old and die,
feeling contented."
(Lao Tzu, *Tao Te Ching*, Chapter 80)

"Therefore, we focus on the present moment,
doing what needs to be done,
without straining and stressing.

To end our suffering,
we focus on the present moment,
instead of our expected result.
So, we follow the natural laws of things."
(Lao Tzu, *Tao Te Ching*, Chapter 63)

## (5) The Natural Cycle

TAO says that everything in life must follow the natural cycle, whether you like it or not, and that you must be patient because nothing is within your control, especially your fate and destiny.

"That which shrinks
Must first expand.
That which fails,
Must first be strong.
That which is cast down
Must first be raised.
Before receiving, there must be giving.
This is called perception of the nature of
things.
Soft and weak overcome hard and strong."
(Lao Tzu, *Tao Te Ching*, Chapter 36)

Spontaneity is the essence of the natural cycle. What goes up must eventually come down; life begets death; day is always followed by night—just like the cycle of the four seasons.

> "Allowing things to come and go,
> following their natural laws,
> we gain everything.
> Straining and striving,
> we lose everything."
> (Lao Tzu, *Tao Te Ching*, Chapter 48)

Intuition of spontaneity is an understanding of the impermanence of all things: nothing lasts no matter how much you strive to keep the impermanent permanent, and everything remains only with that present moment.

> "Strong winds come and go.
> So do torrential rains.
> Even heaven and earth cannot make them last forever."
> (Lao Tzu, *Tao Te Ching*, Chapter 23)

## (6) No Judgment and No Separation

According to Lao Tzu, one should not judge others, nor should one separate oneself from others, because we are all connected, a part of the universe, originating from the same source, which is nothingness, and into nothingness we shall all return.

> "The Creator gives birth to all beings,
> nourishes and cherishes them,
> instructs, comforts, and matures them,
> and then returns them to their origin."
> (Lao Tzu, *Tao Te Ching*, Chapter 51)

Being non-judgmental holds the key to attaining balance and harmony in a world of chaos and disharmony.

"The more we understand the Way,
the less we need to convince others.
Those, who speak much,
know little about the Way."
(Lao Tzu, *Tao Te Ching*, Chapter 56)

## (7) No Picking and No Choosing

Following the natural cycle of all things, you do not need to pick and choose. Picking and choosing is only a sickness of the mind: the futility in striving to control what is essentially uncontrollable.

"People naturally avoid loss and seek gain.
But with all things along the Way,
there is no need to pick and choose.
There is no gain without loss.
There is no abundance without lack.
We do not know how and when
one gives way to the other.

So, we just remain in the center of things,
trusting the Creator, instead of ourselves.
This is the essence of the Way."
(Lao Tzu, *Tao Te Ching*, Chapter 42)

Picking and choosing is synonymous with control of self, others, and everything around, which is against the basic laws of nature.

"Controlling external events is futility.
Control is but an illusion.
Whenever we try to control,
we separate ourselves from our true nature.
Man proposes; the Creator disposes.
Life is sacred: it flows exactly as it should.
Trusting in the Creator, we return to our breathing,
natural and spontaneous, without conscious control.

In the same manner:
sometimes we have more,
sometimes we have less;
sometimes we exert ourselves,
sometimes we pull back;
sometimes we succeed,
sometimes we fail.

Trusting in the Creator, we see the comings and goings of things,
but without straining and striving to control them."
(Lao Tzu, *Tao Te Ching*, Chapter 29)

TAO wisdom is to embrace *all*, instead of picking and choosing this and that.

"Good fortune and misfortune are all in one.
Seeking one and rejecting the other,
we become completely confused.
Striving for goodness and righteousness,
we become evil and wicked."
(Lao Tzu, *Tao Te Ching*, Chapter 58)

TAO wisdom, however, does not imply that there is no free will or freedom of choice.

> "Fame or self, which is dearer?
> Self or wealth, which is greater?
> Gain or loss, which is more painful?
>
> Accumulating or letting go, which causes more suffering?
> Looking for status and security, we find only suffering.
> Knowing our true nature, we find joy and peace.
> With nothing lacking, the whole world belongs to us."
> (Lao Tzu, *Tao Te Ching*, Chapter 44)

Embracing everything is beneficial because it holds the key to enlightenment, which is the understanding of what TAO is all about.

> "The Way to the Creator has no blueprint.
> With faith and humility, we seek neither pride nor blame.
> Our actions then become righteous and impeccable.
> Our lives are illumined with the Creator's light.
>
> Everything that happens to us is beneficial.
> Everything that we experience is instructional.
> Everyone that we meet, good or bad, becomes our teacher or student.

We learn from both the good and the bad.
So, stop picking and choosing.
Everything is a manifestation of the mysteries
of creation."
(Lao Tzu, *Tao Te Ching*, Chapter 27)

## (8) No Expectation and No Over-doing

TAO emphasizes "wu-wei" (無為): "Wu" (無) literally means "no" and "wei" (為) means "doing." Due to the literal translation of the original text, "wu-wei" is sometimes misinterpreted as "non-doing," and even regarded as a "passive" way of looking at life by Lao Tzu. "No over-doing" is a more appropriate translation of "wu-wei."

Contrary to conventional wisdom, which focuses much on effort, TAO wisdom emphasizes "effortless" effort.

"The softest thing in the world
overcomes what seems to be the hardest.

That which has no form
penetrates what seems to be impenetrable.

That is why we exert effortless effort.
We act without over-doing.
We teach without arguing.

This is the Way to true wisdom.
This is not a popular way
because people prefer over-doing."
(Lao Tzu, *Tao Te Ching*, Chapter 43)

"We act without over-action.
We manage without interference.
We enjoy without attachment.

Effrontery is just
an opportunity for loving-kindness.
Great accomplishments are only
a combination of small steps.
Difficult tasks are no more than
a series of easy steps."
(Lao Tzu, *Tao Te Ching*, Chapter 63)

## (9) Humility and the Ego

If TAO wisdom could be summarized in one word, it is the word "humility."

Humility is the enemy of the ego, while pride is its best friend. With humility, you see who you really are, and not who you think or wish you were. With humility, you become harmonious with the Creator, who provides you with the profound wisdom to live in this material world. Harmony is an achievement, and not a free gift from the Creator.

"Focusing on status gives us pride, and not humility.
Hoarding worldly riches deprives us of heavenly assets."
(Lao Tzu, *Tao Te Ching*, Chaper 3)

"Heavenly grace is like a well of water,
free to all, just for the asking.
It is inexhaustible: the bounty of eternal life.
It quenches all human thirst:

the thirst for anger, desires, and vengeance.
Thirsty no more, we find peace and heavenly
grace."
(Lao Tzu, *Tao Te Ching*, Chaper 4)

"Ever humble, we see the mysteries of all
things created.
Ever proud, we see only the manifestations of
all things created.

Only the mysteries, and not the manifestations,
show us the Way to true wisdom."
(Lao Tzu, *Tao Te Ching*, Chaper 1)

Living in this world of depression, we have no way out
or through, but only *through* TAO, which is the Way.

# FIVE

# THE WAY "THROUGH" DEPRESSION

## (1) The Bag and Baggage

Life journey is forever on a long and winding road with many detours and sideways. On this bumpy life journey, we all carry with us our own bag and baggage, containing our individual beliefs, feelings, and skills, some of which may ultimately become the signs and symptoms of our own depression.

Thinking questions

- What are you carrying in your own bag and baggage?
- Who packed your bag and baggage? Did others help you with your packing or unpacking?
- How long have you been carrying your own bag and baggage?
- Is your own bag and baggage getting heavier with each day passing?
- Does your own bag and baggage serve the purpose of your life journey in any way?
- Have you ever thought of unpacking some, if not all, of what is inside your own bag and baggage?

What is inside an individual's bag and baggage could be anything from anger, bitterness, frustration, regret, sadness, shame, to "what-if"—the major components of depression.

TAO is the human wisdom, which is the Way of going *through* what is in your bag and baggage.

## (2) TAO and Enlightenment

TAO and enlightenment are two separate and different entities.

First of all, TAO is the Way *through* anything and everything you encounter and experience in your life. It is a pathless path to the understanding that its purpose is not to get you *to* any particular place or a specific goal. It is just a journey of your own self-discovery and self-understanding. By the same token, TAO does not show you how to avoid or get out of your depression; it only helps you go *through* your depression so that you may or may not become enlightened by those experiences.

Enlightenment is self-awakening, or attaining a very different way of looking at everything with totally new perspectives. Humans live by the eternal law of cause and effect: that is, if you do something good, you will get a good result; if you do something bad, you will then get a bad result. Enlightenment is self-awakening to the unique consciousness that an individual experiences regardless of what has taken place. Simply put, you just let yourself experience *both* the good and the bad, or just about *anything* in your life; going *through* those experiences may or may not change your own perspectives, but that is not the point. Enlightenment is not a state of mind that you can force yourself into; it may or may not even come, but that is irrelevant and unimportant—just *experience* whatever that comes along your way.

**The Ultimate Truth:**

> "I used to see mountains as mountains, and waters as waters. When I arrived at a more intimate knowledge, I came to the point where I saw that mountains are not mountains, and waters are not waters. But now that I have got its very substance, I am at rest. For it is just that I see mountains once again as mountains, and waters once again as waters."
> **Ching Yuan**

> "As to reaching the other shore, if one reaches it, one is not reaching the other shore. Both not reaching it, and *not* not-reaching it are really reaching. This shore means birth and death; the other shore means *Nirvana* (enlightenment)."
> **Tao Sheng**

TAO gets your *through* your depression, but it may or may not get you out of it; TAO may give you the understanding of *how* and *why* you might have your depression, but it does not necessarily enlighten you with the wisdom to get out of it.

If you become enlightened, you will look at your own depression quite *differently*, because TAO has led you *through* it. On the other hand, if you do not become enlightened after going *through* your depression, it is okay too because *that* is TAO. Just *experience* it; whether it enlightens or does not enlighten you is irrelevant and unimportant—just as Ching Yuan said, you will see "mountains once again as mountains, and waters once again as waters"; or according to Tao Sheng, "both not reaching it, and *not* not-reaching it are really reaching" because they are just words, which are only symbols, no more and no less. TAO is beyond the power of words, which themselves cannot describe TAO, except guiding you *towards* TAO and then let you experience everything in your life in a totally different way.

## (3) The Ego and the Human Flaw

You may think you have many life obligations, such as taking care of your loved ones, your family, your career, and among others. But there is only one true life obligation you must focus on: being who you really are.

We are all created to be in this world for only one purpose: to be our true self, and not to be what and who we wish we were. Conventional wisdom tells us to find our role model, pursue our life goals based on that role model. Subconsciously, we may all begin to dream that we are someone else that we are not. That is *how* we have all created an ego-self for ourselves.

The truth of the matter is that we *all* have an ego-self, and that is why we *all* have depression, without any exception. The human ego is the underlying cause or source of human depression. Unfortunately, the human ego is also the human flaw responsible for most of the problems and troubles that we are all facing, and that human flaw inevitably and ultimately leads to our own depression.

The reality is that we cannot get rid of our ego because that is our uniquely individual identity. That said, we can somehow diminish it, or at least not let it get out of control and dominate us eventually. Remember, the size of your ego-self is directly proportionate to the intensity of your depression.

Your identity is neither a social security number nor just

a face. Your identity is your *inner self* or your *self-worth* as a person that you perceive. Many people strive to build their identities by manipulating *acceptance* and *attention* from others. Sadly, that often times does not work: your true identify should be based on how *you* perceive yourself, rather than on how you perceive what *others* may think of you. In addition, your true identity should not be built upon your own inflated ego.

Your sense of self-worth is directly related to how things are going, how well you are doing, and how much you are getting in your life.

## (4) Emotions and Feelings

Emotions and feelings are two sides of the same coin; they are closely related, but they are two very different things in that the former create biochemical reactions in the body, affecting the physical state, while the latter are mental associations and reactions to the former.

Depression involves the numbing of strong emotions and feelings, especially anger, fear, and shame, that an individual often experiences and carries in his or her own bag and baggage.

According to the Traditional Chinese Medicine (TCM), we all have *qi* (氣), which is the internal life-giving energy circulating within each of us, giving us internal balance and harmony. Emotions are energy states too, which may either contribute to or deplete our own internal life-giving energy, causing harmony or disharmony, and leading to positive or negative emotions and feelings.

### The Seven Emotions

According to the Traditional Chinese Medicine, there

are seven emotions that are the underlying causes of many internal diseases, and they are *anger, anxiety, fear, fright, joy, sadness,* and *worry.* Because Chinese medicine is all about internal balance and harmony, these seven emotions may even affect different human body organs. For example, excessive anger impairs the liver, causing headaches, while excessive joy dysfunctions the heart, leading to mania and mental disorders.

Generally speaking, any "excessive" emotion or feeling may trigger insomnia and loss of appetite, which are some of the common symptoms of depression.

## *Anger*

Anger or rage is an ineffective and inefficient way to resolve any issue or make any problem go away. It is a negative emotion that may lead to depression, if it is not properly addressed.

### An illustration

**Donna Alexander**, the creator of the "Anger Room" in Chicago, first thought of the idea as a teenager living in Chicago. Having witnessed much domestic violence and many conflicts at school as a teenager, Donna Alexander finally decided to create a space where anyone can lash out without serious consequences. While at the "Anger Room," the guests, after paying a fee, are given a safe space to unleash their anger and rage by smashing and destroying objects, such as glasses or even a TV. In addition, the room can also be set up to look like an office or a kitchen, where anger often becomes totally uncontrollable.

### Thinking questions

Can you *really* hold off your anger until *after* you have checked in at the "Anger Room"?

If you are so accustomed to smashing and destroying many objects at the "Anger Room," could you still *restrain* yourself from doing the same when your anger is sudden and unmanageable in the office or the kitchen?

The reality

As much as 50 percent of human diseases may be psychosomatic. Therefore, it is not an overstatement that the mind and diseases are interconnected.

**Dr. Caroline B. Thomas**, M.D., of John Hopkins School of Medicine, discovered that cancer patients often had a prior poor relationship with their parents, attesting to the pivotal role of emotions in the development of cancer. In another study by **Dr. Richard B. Shekelle** of the University of Texas School of Medicine, it was found that depression patients were not only more cancer prone but also more likely to die of cancer than the other patients. If emotions play a pivotal role in cancer, by the same token, negative emotions may also adversely affect the symptoms or the prognosis of any human disease. Thoughts of anger, despair, discontent, frustration, guilt, or resentment are instrumental in depressing the physiological processes, including the human body's immune response—a formula for promoting the development of an autoimmune disease.

According to other studies, strong negative emotions, such as anger, can create destructive mental energy that is health damaging. However, it must be pointed out that it is more damaging in *not* experiencing raging anger, or *not wanting* to experience it than in actually experiencing it. The former may cause diseases, or trigger a depression.

## Another illustration

Near the end of 2016, a road rage occurred in Arkansas, ending in the death of a 3-year-old boy.

A woman, with her 3-year-old grandson sitting at the back of her car, stopped at a stop sign. A man in the car right behind honked her, and the woman honked back; the road rage then began with the man firing a gun shot at the woman's car, and ended in tragedy.

## Reflective thoughts

What could possibly be going on in the mind of the aggressor and that of the victim at the stop sign right before the tragedy?

It could have been: "You're in my way, dude!"; "I've as much a right as you do to be where I am!"; "Get the hell out of my way!"; "How dare you honk me! Who do you think you are?"

## Thinking questions

What would *you* have done, if you were the man in the car?

What would *you* have done, if you were the woman in the car?

## Conventional wisdom

Conventional wisdom is to use *distraction* to defuse and dissipate the sudden anger or rage.

**Thomas Jefferson** famously said, "When angry, count 10, before you speak; if very angry, 100."

## TAO wisdom

According to TAO, take a deep breath, review the situation, and ask yourself one simple question: what is the original purpose of driving your car—to get to your destination, or to get angry?

Don't hold your anger in; instead, let it go, by breathing it out. Don't let it go as pain; instead, let it go as your *acceptance*. Don't let your acceptance be viewed as a sign of your own weakness; instead, let it be a statement of your own communication to yourself that getting to your destination is much more important than getting angry.

Remember, anger is always present to serve a purpose to release some deeper issues, problems, and internal conflicts that you may be carrying in your own bag and baggage all these years. It is always better to release anger than to turn it around to destroy yourself. Suppressing anger, on the other hand, is also self-destructive, as the negative energy redirects itself back into your own body. Anger in itself is always a path of destruction no matter what. Resolve anger by developing habits that may release internal conflicts in a constructive manner before it can be released as rage.

Remember, the world always reflects your actions. If you lash out in rage, then the world lashes back at you with that same rage causing pain or grief that still has to get resolved. There is no true "release" of anger, except by resolution.

TAO teaches that peace is the true warrior's path. The sword while an option is never used with anger, or you may have lost from the start. According to **Lao Tzu**, "The best fighter is never becoming angry."

Learn to do the following when you become angry:

- Take a deep *diaphragm breath* (See **Appendix B**), and just feel your anger as you breathe in.
- Look at your anger in your mind.
- Accept that you are *now* angry, and then slowly release your anger as you breathe it out.
- If necessary, use your arm like a sword to sweep away your anger and cut through your feelings of anger, while saying: "I can see my anger: it *is* as it *was.*"

Subconsciously, we all exert a great deal of mental energy to hold on to the past, which is no more than what we *think* happened. In the *now*, what happened in the past is just a memory, and no longer there; all memories are no longer truths, but at best only guidelines for the future. That is to say, your anger *is* as it *was.* Just learn to release your anger over any issue. Anger on its own has no power at all, except the power you give it to make it *real* to you.

The bottom line: anger is often caused by an inflated ego that one has to be right about an issue; without an ego, nothing can anger or trouble you. Seek only your internal balance and harmony.

"We do not become aggressive when we are confronted.
We do not become angry when we are provoked.
We see neither an enemy nor a competitor, because we do not seek our own way.

Knowing both our strengths and weaknesses, we use them to complement one another.
Thus, we find balance and harmony.

Naturally and easily, we follow the Way."
(Lao Tzu, *Tao Te Ching*, Chapter 68)

Just do not let your anger depress you!

## *Joy and sadness*

The emotion of joy, in particular *excessive* joy, may, surprisingly, lead to depression. It is not uncommon that many people experience winter blues right after the joyful celebration of Christmas and the New Year.

<u>TAO wisdom</u>

What goes up must also come down; any excess is always followed by depletion, and therefore damaging. *Moderation* holds the key to attaining balance and harmony.

> "With the golden mean, there is moderation.
> With moderation, our limits are unknown.
> With unknown limits, our potentials are infinite.
> With infinite potentials, our power is everlasting.
> With the golden mean, we accommodate ourselves to
> the ever-changing world around us.
> We simplify the complicated with gentle ease,
> like a mother caring for her child."
> (Lao Tzu, *Tao Te Ching*, Chapter 59)

## *Anxiety, fear, fright, and worry*

All negative emotions, in excess, may lead to depression. For example, if people over-praise you, your ego may become inflated; and you may then subconsciously develop fear—fear of not getting more praise, or fear of not living up to the praise. Conversely, if people criticize you, you may also develop distress to overcome the disgrace from the criticism.

Of all human emotions, *worry* is perhaps the least useful and serves no purpose at all, except causing unnecessary anxiety and developing a depressive mood. The problem with worry is that it focuses on an imaginary future.

TAO wisdom

According to **Lao Tzu**, "Care about what other people think and you will always be their prisoner."

Seeking success and avoiding failure are no more than pride and fear; they are only expressions of the human conditions erroneously perceived by the human mind.

> "Success is avoiding failure; avoiding failure is seeking success.
> Both originate from fear and pride: the source of human suffering."
> (Lao Tzu, *Tao Te Ching*, Chapter 13)

According to TAO, everything follows the natural order of things; that is, everything is in its proper place and will work out the way it is supposed to work out, irrespective of your worrying and regardless of your deliberate interference to make things happen the way you want them to happen.

Remember, worrying will never change the outcome. According to **Lao Tzu**, if you water your dreams with worry and fear, you will produce weeds; if you water your dreams with optimism and solutions, you will cultivate growth and success. Remember, you manifest not what you want but who you are, what you think, and what is deep within you.

> "Centering ourselves in the Creator,
> we have neither fear nor worry.
> It is not that they no longer exist,
> but that they no longer have power over us.
> So, they diminish and disappear from our lives."
> (Lao Tzu, *Tao Te Ching*, Chapter 60)

## All in all

Given the critical role of emotions and feelings in disease development, including depression, always evaluate your negative emotions and feelings, and understand how your thinking mind can control and even change them.

> "Vengeance and violence
> are not along the Way to the Creator,
> no matter how justified they may be.
> Faced with vengeance and violence,
> remember the Creator's precepts:
> forgive our enemies;
> love our neighbors as ourselves.
>
> An eye for an eye
> makes us become what we hate.
> Knowing this, we do not
> rejoice in victory over our enemies,
> nor take delight in their downfall."
> (Lao Tzu, *Tao Te Ching*, Chapter 31)

## (5) Love and Marital Relationships

### Love Recipes

"Love" is a big word in all human civilizations. For all religious disparities, love still plays an essential role in all the religions of the world. Love plays an important role in human lives, especially living in a world of conflicts and aggression.

What is the real meaning of "love"? Love involves our emotions and feelings. We all love some things and some people. Love, ironically enough, gives us both happiness and unhappiness. When the love is fulfilled, we feel happy; when the love is rejected or unrequited, we then feel pain, which becomes the unhappiness. This, unfortunately, is the reality of love.

Loving others is not that easy, and loving yourself is sometimes even more difficulty. This is also the reality of life.

The truth of the matter is that to *truly* love someone is very difficult, if not impossible, unless you love yourself *first*.

### *Self-acceptance*

In a general sense, *self-esteem* is the positive or negative evaluative perception of self. It is a rating of self based on a partial assessment of current and/or past traits. Many mental health professionals claim that achieving higher self-esteem is the keystone of good mental health, in particular, in avoiding depression; such claims, however, are dubious at best.

Low self-esteem is *self-doubt*, often expressed in not

asserting oneself in public or workplace, and not pushing past one's comfort zones.

To love yourself is *self-acceptance*, which is accepting who and what you really are—and not who and what you wish you were (that is, your ego-self). It should also be pointed out that "loving yourself" and "loving your ego-self" are not quite the same. The former is loving yourself for who you really are despite all your imperfections; the latter involves loving or craving to be the person you wish you were. "Loving yourself" means you can love others as well because they are not very different from you in that they, too, are as imperfect as you are. On the other hand, "loving your ego-self" means it is very difficult to love others because you want to distinguish and separate yourself from others; accordingly, others must somehow satisfy your ego *first* before you can love them. That explains why if you have a big ego-self, you cannot easily and readily love others.

The bottom line: if you can accept yourself as who and what you are, then it may become much easier for you to accept and love others as who and what they are.

## The oneness of all life

Accepting and loving others implies having mindfulness of the inter-connection between people; that is to say, no man is an island, according to the famous British poet **John Donne**. This mindfulness leads to love, and then to the awareness of the presence of God or that of a Higher Being. Love is the *first* step towards spirituality.

The oneness of all life is one of the basic laws of Nature: that is, we are all interconnected with one another. This universal moral principle holds the key to true and lasting freedom in living. Without that freedom, we are forever living in human bondage that inhibits further development of the wellness of the body, the mind, and the soul. Without this wellness alignment, there is no wellness wisdom.

## An illustration

A pastor from Hong Kong was invited to give a sermon in China. A woman from the congregation asked the pastor if it was right to give money to get her son into an elite school. The pastor replied by saying: "Your son getting into that elite school would also imply depriving another child of that same opportunity you are seeking for your child."

A year later, the pastor met the same woman, who told him that her son had got into that elite school but without using her *kwanxi* or connection. The pastor then said to her: "See, God is in control; if you would just let Him."

## Thinking question

If you were the woman with the money and the *kwanxi*, would *you* have done differently?

## Another illustration

In 2012, a Chinese couple from Hong Kong filed a lawsuit against an education consultant in the United States for $2 million dollars, who promised that he could, but did not, get their two sons into Harvard University.

## Application of the oneness of all life

Using "improper" but maybe still perfectly "legal" means to get their two sons into Harvard University might have deprived the opportunities of two other students who might otherwise have been admitted.

A friend of mine had been working for a big corporate company for many years, where he rose to the top because he was honest and hardworking. Some years ago, that corporate company failed, and he was out of employment for some time. Then one day, he accidentally ran into his former boss, who then introduced him to a community college in another state, where he got an administrative position. Without the former *kwanxi* or connection, he would not have got that job based on his previous business background. My friend worked hard, earned his Ph.D., and became the dean of that community college within a few years. That illustrates the positive aspects of *kwangsi* and the oneness of all life too.

Understanding the oneness of all life may further make you realize that you are not different from others, and that we all have our different or similar imperfections, not to mention having the same dreams and desires. That may make it easier for you to accept others and to love them as you love yourself. Love and compassion are expressions of the oneness of all life—a mental attitude that liberates human bondage from the ego-self, which always aims at distinguishing and separating self from others.

## TAO wisdom

Focus on your *connectedness* to others, instead of on your own individual desire to satisfy your ego-self. Remember, every person has a heart, and every heart has a place to love and to be loved, as well as to be connected to other hearts.

Avail yourself of every opportunity in life to express your love and care to others. You pass through life only once, so show your love *now*, and not later.

"The greatest virtue of all is to be unaware of a separate self at all.
Awareness of a separate self makes us want to become valuable.
Not becoming valuable, we tend to hate the separate self.
Hating the separate self, how can we value anyone else?

Freedom from the ego-self, we are free to act without the desire to be valuable.
As a result, everything is done, and people all say: 'It happened *naturally*.'"
(Lao Tzu, **Tao Te Ching**, Chapter 17)

## Empathy and sympathy

Love begins with the recognition of the oneness of all life. With increasing intensity, it may develop into empathy and sympathy.

Empathy is much more than sympathy. It is a deep understanding of the painful experiences of another individual that are as meaningful as those of our own because either we have experienced them ourselves, or we can somehow realistically put ourselves in that individual's shoes. Sympathy, on the other hand, is merely our own acknowledgment of another individual's tragic and traumatic emotional feelings, as well as an offering of our own comfort and assurance.

Although empathy is inherent human goodness, it may not be easily expressed due to lack of courage. In addition, it is often much easier to display sympathy than empathy.

The explanation is that sympathy involves only an *understanding* of another individual's problems, such as what it is like to be poor or to be abused, while we may still somehow *distance* ourselves from that individual; but empathy, on the other hand, involves *feeling* that individual's heart in our own hearts and *seeing* that individual's problems with our own eyes. Empathy is not a natural human habit; it has to be cultivated and developed before it can exist in the human heart and mind.

## An illustration

There was a Jewish story of a man who died and was shown two images in both heaven and hell, in which people were sitting at both sides of a long table with a meal before each of them. He noticed that the people in hell were starving, because each of them had a spoon that was much too long to fit into his or her own mouth. However, the people in heaven were well fed, because each was using the same long spoon to feed the person *across* the table.

## *Compassion and loving-kindness*

Compassion means "suffering together." Essentially, it is an emotion or a feeling that arises when you are confronted with another individual's suffering, and you feel motivated to relieve the suffering from that individual.

Loving-kindness is an act of kindness, motivated by love, and expressed to your fellow human beings. Loving-kindness is expressed in human behavior. To optimize this behavior, develop the mindset for love and care, which should become a habit or second nature to you.

## Reflective thought

When a person is not nice to you, what would be your immediate response and reaction to that person? Maybe your mind may tell you: "I won't let him or her step over me like that!" Over time, your natural response will become habitual and spontaneous—a natural way of expressing your individuality and your own rights. In other words, it has become your mindset.

Showing loving-kindness is not about "an eye for an eye," nor is it about your "rights" as an individual. Loving-kindness is an act of love that you *consciously* express to another individual simply because that individual has the same desire to be happy and to avoid suffering, just like yourself. Accordingly, your response is a *reflection* of your love for that individual, irrespective of the behavior of that individual towards you. However, that does not imply that you accept, approve, or even condone the inappropriate behavior of that individual. Loving-kindness is a response in your attempt to *change* the inappropriate behavior of that individual. The outcome of your attempt to change that individual, however, does not affect your own response, because the attempt is out of your compassion and love for that individual, irrespective of your success or failure in *changing* the behavior of that individual.

## Biblical wisdom

Loving-kindness is tantamount to what **Jesus** said about "loving your neighbor" and "turning the other cheek."

> You have heard that it was said, 'Love your neighbor and hate your enemy.' But I tell you, love your enemies and pray for those who persecute you, that you may be children of

your Father in heaven. He causes his sun to rise on the evil and the good, and sends rain on the righteous and the unrighteous.
(**Matthew** 5: 43-45)

But I tell you, do not resist an evil person. If anyone slaps you on the right cheek, turn to them the other cheek also.
(**Matthew** 5: 39)

## Conventional wisdom

**Dalai Lama**, the Tibetan spiritual leader, demonstrates how he instantly connects to people of different cultures, religions, and perspectives.

According to Dalai Lama, on the very first meeting with any individual, he trains himself to feel that the individual is simply "a fellow human being with the same desire to be happy and to avoid suffering as myself." With this oneness-of-all mindset, Dalai Lama then becomes "connected" to everybody, without any exception, and thus showing his loving-kindness.

With awareness, you can develop a positive mentality towards not only yourself but also others—which can improve human relationships by expressing compassion and loving-kindness. Can *you* do just that?

**C.S. Lewis**, author and intellectualist, shows how you, too, can "discipline" your negative emotions. When you know you are not going to behave friendly towards another person, *consciously* put on a more friendly manner, such as a big smile, and behave as if you were a much nicer person than you actually are. In a few minutes, you may actually feel and become friendlier towards that person.

Just light up your face with a big smile, and see if it can

*change* your mindset.

## TAO wisdom

> "The Way is great because of its three essentials:
> compassion, humility, and faith.
> With compassion, there is no fear.
> With humility, there is no strife.
> With faith, there is no impossibility. . . . .
>
> Compassion is the root.
> Humility is the stem.
> Faith in the flower."
> (Lao Tzu, ***Tao Te Ching***, Chapter 67)

According to TAO, everything in life happens for a reason, even though you may not know or understand it immediately. The unpleasant events happening to your life, the unpleasant people your encounter everyday—they not only *test* you spiritually but also *teach* you mentally. The raging driver who honks you, the rude passenger who makes racial slurs at you, the domineering co-worker who overpowers you—they are all your teachers who have something for you to learn from. What you need is the compassion and loving-kindness to react positively and not negatively, the humility to learn and not to reject, and the faith to believe that you can benefit not just yourself but also those who are your "teachers" over the long haul.

## *Faith and hope*

Love, compassion, loving-kindness—they are all the

stepping stones to believing in spirituality, which is faith and hope in humanity.

We are now living in a secular society, where science has become the dominant religion. As a result, many people do not believe in the existence of God. Despite the absence of God in their lives, spirituality may still be present in the hearts of many because they still believe that they have a soul, which is essentially an unfathomable spirit that provides the mind of an individual with direction, guidance, and understanding.

For those who believe in God, the soul is the *connection* to their God. This inherent connection is a line of spiritual communication in the form of prayers, moments of self-awakening, and divine inspiration.

For those who do not have a specific religion, but still believe in the control of a Higher Being greater than themselves, the spirit is the deep *understanding* of the inexplicable control and the natural cycle of all things— certain things in life that are beyond human control and understanding; certain things in life that follow a natural cycle or order, such as life is inevitably followed by death.

For those who are non-believers, but decent human beings, the spirit is the *conscience* that can tell them what is right and wrong, and not just following the law and order.

Therefore, in different ways, we *all* demonstrate that we have a spirit, although some of us may consciously or unconsciously separate ourselves from it. The spirit is like a shadow of ourselves: sometimes we see more of it, and sometimes we see less of it, but it is always within us, part and parcel of our being, forever following us wherever we go, whether we like it or not.

Believing in spirituality may give you the miracle of becoming and transformation.

At some point in your life, especially as you continue to

age, you may begin to sense your own incompleteness, your loneliness, your limitations, your disillusions with human vanity, and you may then begin to long for someone or something that can truly fill and satisfy you or your inner longing. In your youth, you might have turned to the physical world to gratify your own needs and wants, such as successful careers, material comforts, and satisfying relationships, among others. At some point in your life, however, you may suddenly realize that your past wayward pursuits were in vain—much like "chasing after the wind" (**Ecclesiastes** 2, 11), and that you have deviated from your conscience and distanced yourself from spirituality or your Creator.

Believing in spirituality not only gives you faith and hope, but also enhances your consciousness of your true self with the deep desire to become wholesome. Becoming is a miracle of transformation of your whole being. Change is external, but transformation is internal. Change requires you to look outside of you; transformation comes from looking inside of you for wisdom and understanding.

"Faith and lack of faith go along with each other.
The first will be the last, and the last will be the first."
(Lao Tzu, *Tao Te Ching*, Chapter 2)

"Living by the Spirit, we choose a simple and humble lifestyle.
We meditate to enhance our spirituality.
We love our neighbors as ourselves.
We express compassion to all.
We speak with truth and sincerity.

We live in the present moment.
We take action only when necessary.

Without much ado or over-doing, we trust the guidance of the Spirit.
In this manner, life flows like water, fulfilling itself and also everything naturally."
(Lao Tzu, *Tao Te Ching*, Chapter 8)

"Focusing on the Creator,
we are open to all of life.
Opening to all of life,
we embrace all with thankfulness for what we get,
with gratitude for not getting what we deserve.
Discovering the true nature of things,
we live with compassion and loving-kindness.
All endings become beginnings, all returning to the Creator."
(Lao Tzu, *Tao Te Ching*, Chapter 16)

## Forgiveness and forgetting

When you are unable to forgive others for the wrongs they have done to you, you carry those negative feelings in your bag and baggage with you wherever you go, making you feel depressed.

As long as people continue to speak or act against you in some way, you will always carry that emotional bag and baggage with you. The reality is that you can never *control* what people may say or do; even avoiding those individuals does not necessarily eradicate your mental stress caused by the memories in that emotional bag and baggage that you have been carrying with you.

## Conventional wisdom

Many philosophies and most religions preach the virtue of forgiveness and the need to constantly practice it in order to get the subsequent reward. However, for some, that practice is never easy; for others, the demand for immediate vengeance well surpasses the future reward.

## TAO wisdom

It is your own sense of self-importance that allows you to hold on to the bag and baggage of neither forgiving nor forgetting.

It is the false human perception that we are separate and different from others that often leads us to our skewed comparisons with others, which in turn inflate our ego-self. With the ego-self under attack, the illusory and imaginary injuries make grudges unforgivable and unforgettable.

> "Vengeance and violence
> are not along the Way to the Creator,
> no matter how justified they may be.
> Faced with vengeance and violence,
> remember the Creator's precepts:
> forgive our enemies;
> love our neighbors as ourselves."
> (Lao Tzu, *Tao Te Ching*, Chapter 31)

## Marital Relationships

"A feeling that is strong one moment and gone the next, cannot be called love." **Kabir**

## Breakups and divorces

The rate of divorce is skyrocketing in the United States, and the U.S. Census estimates about half of marriages end in divorce. According to relationship experts, the number of long-term relationships heading towards separation is now becoming more frequent with a longer lifespan and a growing acceptability of divorce by our society. What some experts are saying is that people divorce because they have a longer lifespan, and that divorce is no longer a social taboo.

The breakups of couples married for several decades are "cold divorces," often characterized by disengagement, distance, and isolation. These kinds of divorces are often the products of a gradual buildup. The problems may have festered to the point where no one cares any more.

Marriage counselors say that there are benchmarks in a typical marriage where divorce is more apt to occur.

First, divorces often happen during the initial two years of a marriage when the expected honeymoon period is replaced with the reality of having to get accustomed to each other's attitudes and living habits. A second point for divorces is around the five-year to the seven-year mark, where children are typically born. Divorces can also happen when the kids leave their parents' homes. Many empty nesters divorce because they no longer have their children holding them together.

**Pepper Schwartz**, professor of sociology at the University of Washington, one said: "Staying in exactly the right relationship to one another is a very hard thing to maintain every decade. People think you only get closer over time, but that's not necessarily true."

The bottom line: failed relationships are painful, often causing depressive episodes and mood disorders.

<u>Thinking questions</u>

Is marriage like a dress that you throw away when it no longer fits you? If you find that your body has outgrown the dress, can you slim down so that you can fit into the dress again, or can you have it altered so that it can fit into you once again? Is getting a new dress easier than fixing the body or altering the dress? If life is all about changes, then so is marriage. Can you adapt yourself to these changes in order to make it more challenging and interesting, instead of taking a totally different pathway?

The bottom line: you do not just walk away from a marriage because you do not like it anymore. A marriage is a lifetime commitment for thick and thin, for better and for worse.

> "Haven't you read," he replied, "that at the beginning the Creator 'made them male and female,' and said, 'For this reason a man will leave his father and mother and be united to his wife, and the two will become one flesh'? So they are no longer two, but one flesh. Therefore what God has joined together, let no one separate."
> (**Matthew** 19: 4-6)

## *Being and giving*

Love is a gift, but you must be ready to receive it. Surprisingly, many people are just not ready—not only to give away the gift but also to receive it. They come to love with many expectations; love hurts and turns itself into pain when the expectations are unfulfilled. Depression is a mental strife to avoid or to confront that emotional pain from a failed and unfulfilled love relationship.

TAO wisdom

According to TAO, *real* love does not hurt because it is about *being* and *giving*, and not about *feeling* and *receiving*. That is, *being* the person not having to use another person in order to make you feel better or good about yourself. Love is not about your feelings, but about your *doing*—giving away your free gift of love. The reality is that true love is neither conditional nor based on someone or something else; it is simply an act of *giving* in the form of a gift. With no expectation, genuine love does not hurt, but infatuation that depends on others' response always hurts.

## *Fearing and rejecting*

> There is no fear in love; perfect love drives out
> all fear.
> (**1 John** 4: 18)

A common scenario in failed love relationships is *fear*— fear that you are not "good enough" for that "right" person for the "perfect" love relationship in your mind. That is to say, in your subconscious mind, out of fear that the "perfect" love relationship might not last, you may then begin to "mask" what you do not like about yourself, instead of opening yourself completely and honestly.

Ironically enough, that is *how* many so-called "perfect" love relationships turn sour and end unhappily in self-fulfilling prophecy.

TAO wisdom

According to TAO, nobody is perfect, including you and your partner. If you cannot love yourself *completely* in spite of your shortcomings and imperfections, you will also subconsciously *reject* your partner for the same reasons. It is important that you *accept* the good and the bad in a love relationship; you cannot just take the good and reject the bad. A love relationship is there to tell you what you *need*, and not what you *want*.

A distorted perception of self-worth in an individual is often the underlying cause of depression that causes pain which is real to that individual. The reality is that you may *feel* the pain, but you do not have to *suffer* from it. In life, pain may not be an option, but suffering is often a personal choice. Pain is natural; just learn to *receive* it—that is, experiencing it, instead of explaining or dwelling upon it unnecessarily.

## (6) Human Relationships

The complexity of human relationships is the source of conflicts and unhappiness, often leading to depression. But when you are actually going *through* those depressive experiences, what should you do?

**The Obstacles**

Indeed, there are many obstacles to maintaining good and harmonious relationships in family, in workplace, and in society.

## Internal imbalance and disharmony

According to TAO, if you have any internal imbalance and disharmony, you will see everyone and everything around you a reflection of *you*, or what is *inside* you. Neither is internal peace a myth, nor are internal conflicts a condition of existence. Inner peace is an acquired state of mind that recognizes that conflicts—both internal and external—will arise from time-to-time, and that they are all unstoppable. However, all conflicts can be resolved, and sanctity can be restored.

TAO wisdom

According to **Lao Tzu**, this is how we might lose our internal balance and harmony:

> "Reaching out for it, we fall.
> Running to catch it, we stumble.
> Pretending to become enlightened, we become confused.
> Trying to do it right, we fail.
> Looking for praise, we become disappointed.
> Holding onto it, we lose.
>
> Letting go of straining, striving, and strutting, we find the wisdom in the Creator."
> (Lao Tzu, ***Tao Te Ching***, Chapter 14)

"We do not let ourselves be blown to and fro.

Otherwise, we lose touch with who we really
are;
or, worse, who the Creator is."
(Lao Tzu, **Tao Te Ching**, Chapter 26)

"We experience the Creator in our own true
nature.
If we are one with Him, peace comes upon our
lives,
like soft rain falling from heaven,
like joy rising from the earth,
like a mighty river flowing.
Our world then becomes a paradise,
and natural goodness is written in our hearts."
(Lao Tzu, **Tao Te Ching**, Chapter 32)

So *how* do you have *internal* balance and harmony within
yourself? Just look deep inside you to have a better
understanding of what you really seek in your partner, or
from any other individual. Always use your *consciousness of
breath* to go deep into your inner being. Do some deep
diaphragmatic breathing (See **Appendix B**) to give yourself
a sense of internal peace and harmony. Just be conscious of
breathing like a baby.

Conscious of breath also opens the door to knowing
yourself. TAO focuses on *quietude* and *spontaneity*, which are
attributes of internal peace and harmony of the body, the
mind, and the spirit. TAO is also about the art of *listening*
with the body, which stops temporarily the thinking mind,
which is the speaker, and thereby creating space between
the speaker and the listener. TAO teaches you to apply the
art of listening to everyday situation by learning to focus on
your breathing when someone is talking; this is how you
may learn to become a better listener.

Breathing is also about focus and deep concentration on the present moment, which is the immediacy of here and now, so as to remove temporarily the "internal dialogue" between your conscious mind and your subconscious mind. Remember, your mind is forever kept busy reminiscing and rummaging through the past, as well as being constantly preoccupied with thoughts anticipating the future.

When the mind is quiet—in absence of the fear of the sound of silence—the mind can then experience clarity of thinking that may enable you to know yourself. If you do not know yourself, how can you know others for who they are and what they want? How often we say someone has an attitude; but do we also have an attitude towards that someone?

So, meet any conflict head on, deal with it, and resolve it, if possible, and proceed on with your life journey. Just remember that the world is full of wondrous variety, a wide array of people and things that you just need to explore and experience so that you may have a better understanding of the complex world that you are now living in.

## Incomplete human knowledge

Human actions, especially negative ones, are based on *knowledge* of self and others, which is often incomplete and inadequate. Many people hardly know themselves. If they do not know their own emotional needs, how would they know the emotional needs of others?

TAO wisdom

Because human knowledge is limited, we should judge neither others nor ourselves.

"The Creator has no judgment, no preference:
He treats everything and everyone alike.
Every manifestation attests to the mysteries of
His creation.

So, we, too, embrace everything and everyone
with no judgment, no preference.
His grace, never depleting and forever
replenishing, shows us the Way.
Judgment and preference separate us from His
grace, causing attachment.
Only with His grace do we find renewal and
rebirth along the Way."
(Lao Tzu, *Tao Te Ching*, Chapter 5)

Always be mindful of the needs of others *first*, instead of
just those of your own, and that is always the Way to go.

## *Incorrect human perceptions*

Human perceptions are based on *attitudes*, *beliefs*, and
*habits*, which are often biased and distorted because they are
based on an individual's unique past experiences. Let go of
your attachments to the past, especially your past negative
emotions and experiences carried in you bag and baggage.
Incorrect perceptions often cause inappropriate actions,
reactions, or lack of actions, and thus damaging human
relationships.

TAO wisdom

"Blessed is he who has no judgment of self and
others.

He will find contentment and empathy in everyone.

Letting go of everything is the Way to the Creator."
(Lao Tzu, *Tao Te Ching*, Chapter 9)

Always be mindful of the possibility of your perceptions of others being incorrect.

## Self-preoccupation

Our culture teaches us not only "self love" but also "self-esteem," which literally means esteeming "yourself." Self-preoccupation fosters the belief that "I am special" or reinforces the "mine-is-better" attitude. The net result is that you now begin to believe whole-heartedly that your convictions *do* carry more weight than those of others.

Always be mindful of your self-centeredness, which is the root cause of bias, prejudice, and non-acceptance of others.

TAO wisdom

Look at Nature, and you will see the reason why it lasts: the reason is that they do not exist for themselves, and that is why they can last forever. So, focus on others, instead of on yourself all the time.

"Blessed is he who has no ego-self.
He will be rewarded with humility to connect with the Creator."
(Lao Tzu, *Tao Te Ching*, Chapter 9)

Focusing on others, you may then see the world quite *differently.*

## Right to express

The American society encourages the "right" to express oneself, including one's emotions. Instead of reigning in your negative emotions, you are entitled to giving vent to all your negative impulses—even at the expense of hurting others' feelings. This undisciplined emotion is the failure to restrain the negative impulses, which often cause human conflict and destroy relationships.

Always be mindful of your own undisciplined negative impulses to express yourself.

TAO wisdom

According to TAO, words mean little.

"The Way is of few words.
Actions speak louder than words. . . .
Why then so much concern over what to say,
or what to do?
Living is but an expression of the life given by
the Creator.
Our true nature is a reflection of that
expression.
Those who are with the Creator, the Creator is
also with them.
So, success and failure are seen as part of a
perfect whole.
Everything is accepted and fully lived
accordingly."

(Lao Tzu, *Tao Te Ching*, Chapter 23)

"Since the beginning of the beginning,
there have been names for everything.
The more words we use,
the more distinctions we make.
The more distinctions we have,
the more we pick and choose.
As a result, we separate ourselves
from our own true nature.

To return to peace and harmony,
we must be like rivers and streams,
returning to their origin—the ocean."
(Lao Tzu, *Tao Te Ching*, Chapter 32)

## The Way Through

Human conflicts are many. The Way is the only way to
go *through* them, rather than avoiding them.

## *Balance and harmony*

Always maintain your internal balance and harmony.
Remember, the world around you is always a reflection of
what is deep inside you.

"The Way is easy,
yet people prefer distracting detours.
Beware when things are out of balance.
Remain centered within the Creator.

Distractions are many,

in the form of riches and luxuries.
They allure us from the Way.
Accumulations are like extortions of the poor.
They bring only disaster and suffering.
Do not deviate from the Way."
(Lao Tzu, *Tao Te Ching*, Chapter 53)

"When there is no desire to be someone that
we are not,
separate from our true nature designed by the
Creator,
all things are in perfect balance and harmony."
(Lao Tzu, *Tao Te Ching*, Chapter 37)

## *The five elements and the natural cycle*

The five elements of the ancient Chinese are: *metal, wood, water, fire,* and *earth.*

The five elements balance and complement one another to create both internal harmony and the natural cycle. To illustrate, water nourishes trees or wood; without wood, there will be no fire (which burns wood); without fire burning wood, there will be no earth (the ashes from the burnt wood); without earth, there will be no metal (from the earth itself); through condensation, fire heats metal to produce water; without metal, there will be no water; without water, there will be no tree or wood.

These five elements are interdependent on one another for their own existence in the natural cycle. In many respects, human relationships and our dealings with one another attest to the cyclical nature of the world we are living in.

TAO wisdom

Think about your own nature with reference to the five elements. Are *you* strong and independent like *metal*, bold and pioneering like *wood*, soft and flexible like *water*, fiery and passionate like *fire*, or nurturing and receptive like *earth*?

Also, think about the different natures of the people around you, or you have to deal with. Understanding their different natures may result in better and more harmonious relationships with them. Indeed, the five elements can give you profound wisdom and insight into many different life situations to help you avoid unnecessary everyday conflicts and disparities.

The bottom line: learn to live a life without any conflict and confrontation with others. To do just that, you need to know not only yourself but also others.

> "Knowing others is intelligence.
> Knowing ourselves is true wisdom.
> Overcoming others is strength.
> Overcoming ourselves is true power."
> (Lao Tzu, ***Tao Te Ching***, Chapter 33)

Everything will be in its natural place because everything follows the natural cycle. So why do you strain, stress, and strut yourself?

> "We stay in the very center of the Creator,
> and refrain from controlling our destiny.
> Everything will evolve and fall into its natural place,
> according to the laws of the Creator."
> (Lao Tzu, ***Tao Te Ching***, Chapter 37)

## *Soft and flexible*

To help you overcome conflicts and resolve issues, you need the flexibility of TAO. Always be flexible, instead of being strong-willed and uncompromising.

"The Way is paradoxical.
Like water, soft and yielding,
yet it overcomes the hard and the rigid.
Stiffness and stubbornness cause much suffering.

We all intuitively know
that flexibility and tenderness
are the Way to go.
Yet our conditioned mind
tells us to go the other way."
(Lao Tzu, ***Tao Te Ching***, Chapter 78)

It does not mean that you let people walk all over you and do nothing. Just step back, giving yourself some open space to create a detached mindset. If you are combative and strike back with a personal attack, you are in fact driving a nail into wood with a hammer; when you pull out the nail, the puncture on the wood is still permanently there. So do not do or say anything that you may regret for the rest of your life. Always defer your anger for later processing.

## All in all

Having good human relationship with others may not only afford you joy and happiness, but also heal you mentally, physically, and spiritually through your own connections with others. On the other hand, having bad human relationships may make you feel sad, lonely, hopeless, and depressed.

> "If we are in harmony with the Creator,
> we are like newborn babies,
> in natural harmony with all.
> Our bones are soft, and our muscles are weak,
> but our grip is strong and powerful."
> (Lao Tzu, *Tao Te Ching*, Chapter 55)

We are all living in a world of speed in which nothing seems to last too long, including human relationships. In contemporary living, there is too much focus on speed. Given that life is short, there is a great deal to be done and accomplished. As a result, you may feel the compression of time, and you may have developed a compulsive mind with a multi-tasking mindset, such as talking and texting on the phone while driving at the same time.

Remember, it is your compulsive mind that makes you feel distressed and unhappy. Ironically, it is because you know and believe that nothing lasts, that you want to do more, much more than necessary, hoping against hope that some of the things that you are doing may last a little longer. Because nothing lasts, so you begin to look for new ones to replace the ones that have expired. An example is a love relationship: if it does not turn out to be what you have expected, you just let it end itself, and then start looking for another one because it is your belief that nothing lasts.

According to TAO, truly nothing lasts, but that is the *wrong* way to look at the impermanence of things. The *right* way is to look at everything with *non-attachment*, which is letting go of whatever that happens in your life, be it joy or sorrow, success or failure, happiness or un-happiness. Letting go essentially means understanding that nothing lasts, and that what goes up must also come down, because everything in life follows the natural order—just like youth becoming old age, and life transforming into death. Understanding the impermanence of all things may change *how* you are going to live your life and interact with others. If nothing lasts, then let go of everything, and live your life to the fullest, which is in the present. The past was gone, so let it go; the future is yet to come, so let go of your expectations. Only the present is real, so live and enjoy it to the fullest.

> "Therefore, we focus on the present moment,
> doing what needs to be done,
> without straining and stressing.
>
> To end our suffering,
> we focus on the present moment,
> instead of our expected result.
> So, we follow the natural laws of things."
> (Lao Tzu, *Tao Te Ching*, Chapter 63)

## (7) Money and Material Comforts

We all want abundance, and not emptiness. We all desire abundance in education, family, relationships, profession, and wealth; nobody wants emptiness—one thing nobody wants in life. But abundance often becomes attachments in our lives. Ironically enough, we need emptiness to attain the ultimate truths of life and living, which is the wisdom in living. To attain this profound human wisdom, we need emptiness—or an empty mind to begin with.

MY WAY! NO WAY! TAO IS THE WAY!

## An Empty Mind

> "Blessed is he who has an empty mind.
> He will be filled with knowledge and wisdom
> from the Creator."
> (Lao Tzu, *Tao Te Ching*, Chapter 9)

First of all, we need an empty mind with reverse thinking to think quite *differently*, and not according to conventional wisdom. Then, we need to become empty *consciously*, which is letting go of all our attachments to the material world we are living in. Attachments are emotional distractions of the mind that prevent clarity of thinking, without which there is no access to the ultimate truths of life and living. Knowing these ultimate truths may enable us to live as if everything is a miracle.

Emptiness is the essence of receiving. Before we can receive, we must let go *first*. Letting go of all attachments to the material world is the first step we all must take. As **Lao Tzu** once said, "A journey of a thousand miles must begin with the first step." So, begin the first step of letting go. According to **Mother Teresa**, it is more blessed to give than to receive. But many of us do not believe in that: instead, at best, we may think we will give out or let go only *after* we have received abundantly.

## Money Wisdom

Letting go is difficult because there is one thing that most of us have overlooked: money wisdom.

Life is all about *living*—it comes with some hard work and simple integrity, but, above all, the wisdom in living. If life is all about *living*—not just about making and spending money—then it is *not* about regrets and dreams. Regrets look back at the past; dreams look forward to the future. Unfortunately, both are *not* within our control. If the value of money is solely based on accumulation of wealth, or the acquisition of material things, then living indeed becomes a labyrinth of regrets and dreams—regrets over the wrong investment decisions in the past, and dreams of the great fortune in the future.

## *Integrity and money*

The real value of money is *integrity*. This is an important quality that can influence your value of money, in particular, all your financial decisions. Integrity is to value what life has to offer, and not the things purchased with money. Integrity is money wisdom. Life has a great deal to offer, and some of the best things in life are free, such as your ability to think, to reason, to learn, and even to remember—these are especially important if you are getting older. Remember, money is a means to an end, but not an end in itself. This is the *real* value of money, as well as money wisdom

Why is integrity important in terms of money?

If a financial problem arises, your integrity will play a critical role. Instead of *reacting* to the problem due to the flawed value of money, integrity will demand you not to leave it to chance. Integrity will demand you not to ignore the problem. Integrity will demand you come up with a practical and feasible plan, a balanced budget, and some necessary action steps to deal with the financial crisis.

Integrity is one of the *core values* in human life. Do not compromise it under any financial situation. If you do, then you will be distorting the real value of money, as well as compromising your money wisdom.

## Love and money

The whole world out there that you see in front of you right now is nothing more than a projection of what you feel inside. Not only is it a projection of your deep feelings, but also your internal energy. Yes, money is energy too, just like you, me, and everything else. Money is an expression of energy of your subconscious mind, building a complex system of money beliefs, such as "money makes the world go round" and "when I have enough money . . . then I'll be very happy."

**Bruce Lipton**, author and cellular biologist, said: "The function of the mind is to create coherence between our beliefs and the reality that we experience. We generally perceive that we are running our lives with our wishes and our desires. But neuroscience reveals a startling fact. We only run our lives with our creative, conscious mind about 5 percent of the time. Ninety-five percent of the time, our life is controlled by the beliefs and habits that are programmed in the subconscious mind."

That can explain why we find ourselves working in jobs that we do not even like due to our subconscious belief that money is *everything* in life.

The reality is that you can have all the money in the world and still be as miserable as sin. The truth of the matter is that it is *love*, rather than money, that actually makes the world go round. Everybody is chasing money, and looking for ways of getting more. But if missing out love, a vital ingredient, making the world go round will only guarantee failure and unhappiness.

## Money and Happiness

"When we are children, we play with toys.

105

When we grow up,
We want the real thing."
**Uchiyama Roshi**

Does money bring happiness? To many, it does,
especially if they have experienced the lack of it!

## *The poor little rich girl*

**Barbara Woolworth Hutton** was one of the wealthiest
women in the world during the Great Depression. She
experienced an unhappy childhood with the early loss of
her mother at age five and the neglect of her father, setting
her the stage for a life of difficulty forming relationships.
Married and divorced seven times, she acquired grand
foreign titles, but was maliciously treated and exploited by
several of her husbands. Publicly, she was much envied for
her lavish lifestyle and her exuberant wealth; privately, she
was very insecure and unhappy, leading to addiction and
fornication. She died of a heart attack at age 66. At her
death, the formerly wealthy Hutton was on the verge of
bankruptcy as a result of exploitation by her husbands, as
well as of her own lavish and luxurious lifestyle.

Barbara Hutton was the unhappy "poor little rich girl"!
She was widely reported in the media, and her story was
even made into a Hollywood movie.

## *Get-rich-quick*

The love of money may entice many people to engage in
many get-rich-quick schemes, high-risk investments, or
compulsive gambling, leading to debts and many financial
disasters in their lives.

There was the story of a fool who was told that to satisfy his hunger, he had to eat four buns; he ended up eating only the fourth bun when he though that the could take a shortcut instead. In real life, you have to work hard to earn your money, just as you have to eat all the four buns to satisfy your hunger, and not just the fourth one.

Buying lottery tickets is also like eating the fourth bun— another get-rich-quick mindset that many people embrace and entertain.

According to some psychology studies, the overall happiness levels of lottery winners spiked when they won, but returned to their pre-winning levels after just a few months when the thrills of winning wore off. In terms of their overall happiness, the lottery winners were neither significantly happier than the non-winners, nor were they happier than they were before their winnings. Research has shown that *affective forecasting*, which is predicting human future emotions, often makes humans *overestimate* the duration of their future emotional reactions.

Having said that, you might *still* think: "I still want to win the lottery, and let me be *un*happy later!"

## TAO wisdom

According to TAO, money is neither positive nor negative; it is all in the human mind.

But how you *make* your money and how you *spend* your money may turn money into something either positive or negative.

To increase your wealth in a positive way, focus on doing what needs to be done, and no more. On the other hand, the more you do to make money, the less focused you become, and the greater are your expectations of the outcome. *That* may ultimately create not only undue stress but also internal disharmony in your life, turning money into something negative, such as depression.

Increasing your wealth, however, does not necessarily mean spending your money proportionately. That is to say, an individual making more money does not have to buy a much bigger house than what that individual actually needs. To illustrate, **Warren Buffet**, the billionaire, has set an excellent example: he is still living in his $31,500 home he bought some decades ago.

Another classic example is **Ann Russell Miller**, a celebrated socialite from San Francisco, also known as **Sister Mary Joseph**. She, who had ten children and nineteen grandchildren, had grown up in luxury and privilege, and had been living a life of incredible wealth. Instead of shopping at Saks Fifth Avenue she used to do for decades—she suddenly decided to give up everything, and became a nun devoted to living in poverty for the rest of her life. That unbelievable event happened more than two decades ago: one day she held a celebrity party in which she announced her incredible decision, and her announcement was widely reported in the media across the United States. Why did she suddenly make such an incredible decision to drastically change her lifestyle? She said she had a calling, a true vocation that was hard to understand for the general public, and even for the close members of her family.

Excessively increasing one's wants often leads to unduly inflating one's ego as well, and thus creating many negative attachments that are often packed in one's own bag and baggage.

The late **Robert Kennedy** once said: "Sometimes I think that the only people in this country who worry more about money than the poor are the very wealthy. They worry about losing it, they worry about how it is invested, they worry about the effect it's going to have. And as the zeroes increase, the dilemmas get bigger."

**Epicurus**, the ancient Greek philosopher, rightly said that to lead a pleasant life one must avoid luxuries and live simply. The explanation is that luxurious living may make you into a *needy* person whose happiness depends on things that not only are impermanent but also are easily lost.

The bottom line: the pleasures of all sensory stimulation are limited and short-lived, whereas the joy of TAO is unlimited and lasting. With less focus on your attachments to the pleasures of the material world, your heart will be more on your spirituality that will provide you with eternal joy.

> "Stop accumulating riches by being smart.
> Heavenly assets are freely available to all."
> (Lao Tzu, ***Tao Te Ching***, Chapter 19)

Thinking questions

- What has love got to do with your money? How does love equate to money from your own perspective?
- Did you do things with money that, in retrospect, did not seem to make much sense? If so, why did that happen? Can you now repack or unpack your bag and baggage?
- Are your core values in alignment with your work and how you earn your money?
- Do you have your priorities straight, and if so, does the way you spend your money support those priorities?

- Do you know the difference between your needs and your wants, and if so, do you take care of your needs first and wants second, or the other way around?
- Do you know how your money is invested, and do those investments support you core values?
- In future, will you still continue to buy the lottery ticket or the Power Ball?

Reflecting on how you have come to where you are right now may help you understand how all these years have built up your complex system of money beliefs in your subconscious mind, or why all your striving and hard work to get that elusive wealth that has always seemed so vitally important to you.

Now is the time to strip away all the "noise" in your life, the worry about debt, the fear of failure, the deeply buried beliefs about unworthiness that obscure the real you, and serve only to resist the flow of life within you.

Now is the time to fully understand that all your imaginary needs are no more than your wants; they are delusional, causing confusion and distress, and they could never be fulfilled anyhow. They are the underlying causes of your depression.

The never-ending cycle of acquisitions leads to clutter, burden, and self-imprisonment. Decrease is the beginning of letting go, which may free you from attachment, fear, and insecurity.

"When there is abundance, there is lacking.
When there is craving, there is discontentment.
Striving for power to control and influence
every aspect of our lives
is the source of our suffering.

> Obsessed with getting and keeping,
> many of us never really live before we die.
>
> Following the Way,
> we must learn to let go."
> (Lao Tzu, *Tao Te Ching*, Chapter 75)

Remember, you came into this world empty-handed, and now you expect to grab and hold on to everything when you leave. Does that make any sense to you? If you think that you would leave what you have to your children and grandchildren, then remember this: they, just like everyone else, have their own destinies that are totally beyond your or their own control.

## Generosity and Gratitude

> One person gives freely, yet gains even more;
>    another withholds unduly, but comes to poverty.
> A generous person will prosper;
>    whoever refreshes others will be refreshed.
> (**Proverbs** 11:24-25)

Love of others is often expressed in generosity. Be generous with your time, your labor, and with what you have. Show generosity to others around you. Form the habit of giving without expecting any credit, recognition, or just anything in return for your generous gesture. If you give with the intent of receiving, you are a "user" and not a *real* "giver."

Generosity does not necessarily involve spending your money. It is not solely based on your economic status or how much money you have, but on your pure intentions of looking out for society's common good and giving from the bottom of your heart. Generosity should reflect your passion to help others who are in need, or who are less fortunate than yourself.

Giving generously is spiritual giving because God is giving. He gave man life itself (**Acts** 17:25), He constantly sustains man by His providential gifts (**Acts** 14:17), and, most significantly of all, He gave His beloved Son so that man may have eternal life (**John**. 3:16; **Romans** 6:23). If God is so generous, so should we all be!

Generosity is an expression of contentment of what one already has. One does not give simply because one has *more*. Generosity comes only from the heart. Generosity will change one's perceptions of life, especially with respect to letting go of all attachments in this material world. Generosity is a necessity, and not an impossibility, in seeking spiritual wisdom.

> 'Bring the whole tithe into the storehouse, that there may be food in my house. Test me in this,' says the Lord Almighty, 'and see if I will not throw open the floodgates of heaven and pour out so much blessing that there will not be room enough to store it. I will prevent pests from devouring your crops, and the vines in your fields will not drop their fruit before it is ripe,' says the Lord Almighty. (**Malachi** 3: 10-11)

Generosity is also an expression of gratitude—grateful for what one already has, and not for getting what one rightly deserves. Gratitude is, therefore, an appreciation of what the Creator has already given and provided. Without gratitude, you tend to focus on your lack, and thus generating depressive thoughts.

TAO wisdom

> "Understanding that we have everything we need,
> we count our blessings.
> Identifying with our own true nature,
> we hold fast to what endures."
> (Lao Tzu, *Tao Te Ching*, Chapter 33)

The opposite of generosity is the obsession with lack of abundance, which plunges an individual into a bottomless pit of insatiable craving, and discontent—the elements of depression. According to TAO, such obsession deprives you of freedom, which is one of the most important attributes of happiness. It is the freedom from any mental obsession. If your mind keeps thinking about regrets and sorrows in the past, or anxieties about the future, you will never be truly happy. People who do that strive to free themselves from their mental bondage with many distractions in life, such as shopping sprees and material comforts, drugs and alcohol, among many others—they have become their ultimate mental attachments, and, ironically enough, also their impediments in their paths to true happiness.

Freedom from focusing on what you do not have holds the key to happiness. Immediately after the tragic death of **Robin Williams**, the celebrated actor and comedian, the media and the public were at a loss as to *why* he committed suicide. Apparently, he had "everything" that most people would desire in their lives—career, fame, money, family, and even relationships. The plausible explanation for his taking his own life is that, instead of focusing on what he already had, maybe Robin Williams focused on what he did not have—it could be something incredibly insignificant to many of us who do not have what he had. That lack of freedom might explain the inexplicable, or why he killed himself.

## (8) Good Fortunes and Misfortunes

Life may be a bed of roses, but always with thorns. Good fortunes and misfortunes exist side by side, and they complement each other. A misfortune is an ingredient that one needs to blend with the other ingredients of life and living. Life will not be wholesome without misfortunes and tragedies, which exist to enable one to appreciate more what life has to offer.

A case in point

There was a Chinese story . . . 塞翁失馬 A man lost his only horse, which ran away one day. His friends comforted him. But he was not upset at all; instead, he said: "That's not a misfortune." A few days later, his horse came back with a stallion. This time, his friends congratulated him on his good fortune. But he said: "What's so good about that?" Later on, his only son rode on the stallion and broke his leg when he accidentally fell from the horse. Once again, his friends comforted him for the misfortune. But he said: "Breaking his leg may not be a misfortune." Indeed, soon after that, a war broke out, and all the young men were drafted into the army, except the man's son with his broken leg. All of them were later annihilated in a fierce battle. The moral of the story: a misfortune may turn itself into a good fortune.

There is a Chinese saying: "A man's destiny cannot be summarized and sealed until nails are put on his coffin's top." So, nothing is set in stone.

## TAO wisdom

According to TAO, willingness to accept your own fate or destiny provides you with inspiration for right conduct. Not accepting is a controlling and manipulative mindset through unbecoming conduct to control your destiny to get what you want in life.

In TAO, there is no such thing as "good luck" or "bad luck." Let go of the negative concept of bad luck, such as "13" and "touch wood," or even the positive thinking of having good luck. Instead, let the natural flow of life move through you, giving you internal power to make the impossible become possible, the difficult become easy. Simplify your life, and get rid of clutters that make you become superstitious. Remember, luck is something that you create for yourself, and that it is an external reality beyond your control, whereas you can always create your own internal reality of peace to overcome any groundless fear responsible for your internal negative energy.

Everything in this material world has meaning only in comparison with one another, and that goes for good luck or bad luck too. Does "Friday the 13th" worry you? Are you getting yourself depressed by thinking of your bad luck in relation to the good luck of others? Go deeper into the core of your being and take control of your own beliefs, and not follow those of others. Fear is only your mental construct.

According to conventional wisdom, winning is always related to conflict: you must fight in order to win, just like in any contest or competition. The bag and baggage that all winners and losers must carry with them is that their net worth and value are solely based on their winning or losing.

TAO, on the other hand, focuses on doing your best in any endeavor. More importantly, it is *you*, and no one else, who will judge your own wins and losses.

> "Everything that happens to us is beneficial.
> Everything that we experience is instructional.
> Everyone that we meet, good or bad, becomes our teacher or student.
>
> We learn from both the good and the bad.
> So, stop picking and choosing.
> Everything is a manifestation of the mysteries of creation."
> (Lao Tzu, *Tao Te Ching*, Chapter 27)

> "We accept all that is simple and humble.
> We embrace the good fortune and the misfortune.
> Thus, we become masters of every situation.
> We overcome the painful and the difficult in our lives.
> That is why the Way seems paradoxical."
> (Lao Tzu, *Tao Te Ching*, Chapter 78)

## (9) Careers and Life Goals

## Careers

### The bag and baggage

To choose a career, to pursue a career, to change a career, or to end a career—they often come with the bag and baggage of the signs and symptoms of depression, such as fear, regret, disappointment, and among others.

## Career choice

### A case in point

A Chinese couple in Canada have a son who wants to pursue a career in the entertainment industry. Their son in his early thirties decided to go to Beijing to learn the Chinese language as a prerequisite of his career pursuit. His parents have opposed to the idea of his living in Beijing, or rather pursuing a career in the entertainment industry.

### The different perspectives

From the parents' perspectives: a really successful career in the entertainment industry is few and far between, especially if it is not pursued at a much younger age.

From the son's perspectives: money, glamour, and quick recognition often come with success in a career in the entertainment industry.

### The ultimate truths

A be-all-and-end-all career based on only one variable, which is money, may not turn out that way.

Any glamorous career is always competitive, but it does not mean it is unachievable at any age. Have an empty mind that everything is doable and achievable irrespective of the age.

Recognition should not be the only primary reason for pursuing any career; rather, passion should be the driving force behind.

Easy success in any human endeavor hurts ultimately, especially a career in the long term, because it does not expand an individual's capacity and capability to deal with problems when they get tough, or to have the persistence to go through them when things do not turn out as expected. Hard-earned success, on the other hand, may prepare an individual for more success in the future through persistence and perseverance.

## The reality

There is no right or wrong in the choice or pursuit of your career; after all, it is *your* career, and others may be looking at your career from their own perspectives.

Follow your *passion*, not people or what they say. Success comes from hard work, and not from wishful thinking. Spend your internal energy pursuing what you want, not defending or explaining why you want it; the latter has to do with your ego. Always ask yourself many self-intuitive questions about *why* and *how* you want to pursue your career goals.

## TAO wisdom

According to TAO, choosing a career is like digging a well. Did you choose the right spot? Have you dug deep enough? If nothing happens according to your expectation, then self-doubt, reinforced by fear and uncertainty, may make you go for another spot. Going for another spot and yet another one may only bring you further frustration and more disappointment.

The bottom line: carefully choose your career, apply persistent effort, and you will find your initial investment of time and effort rewarding. Even if you choose to move on after a while, you will still find it very worthwhile because you have learned something from it. TAO says that giving up is not an admission of defeat or disappointment; rather, giving up is letting go of any resistance when dealing with the chaos of life, and redirecting your energy to a higher purpose.

> "The Way to the Creator is deep-rooted.
> Unmoved, it becomes the source of all movement.
> Stable, it enables us to act without rashness.
>
> "So, whatever we do, we do not abandon our true nature.
> The world around us is riddled with worries and distractions.
> We remain stable, steady, and steadfast."
> (Lao Tzu, *Tao Te Ching*, Chapter 26)

Do not abandon your true nature: be stable, steady, and steadfast when pursuing your career.

## Career advancement

Career advancement involves many new challenges and increasing responsibilities. If this is what you want, it may provide you with satisfaction and motivation to move on with your current career.

On the other hand, if career advancement is not right for you, then you may consider *lateral move* within your organization, that is, changing your daily duties but without increasing your responsibilities.

TAO wisdom

Wanting or not wanting your career advancement is your choice. According to TAO, your choice should not be based on control or power.

"Likewise, our greatness comes
not from our power or control,
but from our own true nature,
which is living as one with the Creator."
(Lao Tzu, *Tao Te Ching*, Chapter 34)

During career advancement, your procrastination may sometimes become an obstacle, causing frustration. **Lao Tzu** said: "A journey of a thousand miles begins with the first step."

"Great accomplishments are only
a combination of small steps.
Difficult tasks are no more than
a series of easy steps."
(Lao Tzu, *Tao Te Ching*, Chapter 63)

So, begin your first step, and one step at a time, but do not overstep yourself.

"Striving to climb the ladder of success,
we may seem smart.
But trusting our Creator,
we find divine guidance,
which is effortless along the Way."
(Lao Tzu, *Tao Te Ching*, Chapter 28)

Climbing a career ladder successfully is never easy and smooth: involvement with argument and aggression is often inevitable. Ambition often comes with an aggressive and domineering personality, often leading to coercion and imposition.

According to TAO, do what you have to do, but without "over-doing" it, which essentially means acting without attachments or expectations, but with effortless efficiency. While climbing your career ladder, neither push someone over nor use any inappropriate means to remove any obstacle that may stand in your way. Career success stems from your contentment, and not your resentment.

> "Resentment breeds more resentment.
> Only contentment leads to contentment.
> True contentment comes from our true nature:
> not from what we do, or how we do;
> neither from our status nor our control.
>
> The Creator is impartial.
> No one is special."
> (Lao Tzu, *Tao Te Ching*, Chapter 79)

In your career advancement, you may find the urge to argue to prove that you are right.

> "The wise learn to succumb, instead of arguing."
> (*Tao Te Ching*, Chapter 81)

Arguing with your co-workers or just anyone else can never bring any worthwhile benefits. When you feel the urge to argue a point with someone, take a deep breath, bite your tongue, and remind yourself that any combat is due to your own ego.

Countering any aggression with aggression is just like fighting fire with fire. According to TAO, when confronted with aggression, neither fight back nor back down; instead, be gentle but firm. The objective is not to humiliate the aggressor but to transform the harm into harmony, and the aggression into peace.

> "So, we advance
> not at the expense of overstepping anyone.
> So, we gain
> not at the expense of making anyone lose.
> So, we accomplish
> not at the expense of straining ourselves.
>
> We have no enemy.
> We love everyone as ourselves.
> We remain in our true nature;
> otherwise, we lose
> the three essentials of the Way,
> and become our own enemy."
> (Lao Tzu, *Tao Te Ching*, Chapter 69)

On the other hand, if you find that you have assumed an aggressive and domineering personality during your career advancement, do remind yourself the wisdom of not expanding your ego at the expense of others, because career success, like anything else, can never sustain itself over the long haul. The reality is that nothing lasts, not even a very successful career.

## Career change

It is never too late to change your career, and be who you are meant to be. But your desire to change your career should be greater than your fear of failure when taking the challenge to change. Remember, the disappointment you feel today may become the strength to face the challenge you encounter tomorrow.

TAO wisdom

According to TAO, always have an empty mind because nothing is set in stone, and change your career without any fear or expectation.

> "Following the conditioned mind, we fear everything.
> Fear is a futile attempt to control things and people."
> (Lao Tzu, **Tao Te Ching**, Chapter 74)

## Career setbacks

Throughout one's lifespan, career setbacks are often times unavoidable. According to TAO, what goes up must also come down. Career setbacks may give an individual a period of shock, denial, and self-doubt. Indeed, many individuals may experience trouble in accepting the realities of career setbacks, and thus adding regret and resentment to their bag and baggage.

TAO wisdom

Learn to accept everything in life as it is. Instead of wasting your internal energy raging against your self-perceived unfair fate in your career, direct it to creating a better reality. To transform that into a reality, an individual must determine why he or she has failed, must explore new paths, and must seize the right opportunity with the right mind. Remember, a career setback may be a springboard to future success.

> "We accept all that is simple and humble.
> We embrace the good fortune and the misfortune.
> Thus, we become masters of every situation.
> We overcome the painful and the difficult in our lives."
> (Lao Tzu, *Tao Te Ching*, Chapter 78)

## Life Goals

Life goals are directives we wish to take in order to meet some of our basic human needs, such as food, shelter, and clothing. Of course, living in the material world in this day and age may include many other things as well. To get these extra things and to stay alive, we all need to set certain common life goals, such as getting an appropriate education, finding a well-paid job, and starting a family, among others. These life goals are instrumental in raising our own standards from just meeting our basic human needs, as well as giving us some pleasures to satisfy our five senses. Life goals are often set to meeting more than just our basic needs.

But how much *more*? Not only our needs may change over time, but also our wants may also increase excessively compared with our basic needs. This disproportionate increase often leads to unduly inflating our ego as well, and thus creating many more attachments that are packed in our own bag and baggage. Therefore, it is important to balance our needs with our wants in the pursuit of our life goals. Life goals have much more to do with *self*, rather than with others and the world around.

The bottom line: life goals, indispensable as they are, can easily create attachments that are often difficult to let go of, leading to depression.

> "The foolish all have goals.
> The wise are humble and stubborn.
> They alone trust the Creator,
> and not the world He created."
> (Lao Tzu, ***Tao Te Ching***, Chapter 20)

## Self-confidence

Not achieving one's life goals inevitably undermines one's self-confidence, which may often lead to despair and depression.

**Diane Sawyer** once said: "Whatever you want in life, other people are going to want it too. Believe in yourself enough to accept the idea that you have an equal right to it."

Yes, you have an equal right to do what you wish to do with any life goal you may have set your mind on, but bear in mind that others may also have the *same* right as you do.

So, you neither compete nor compare with others; you just act with self-confidence to pursue your own life goals.

When you were young, you believed in anything and everything—even in the fairies. However, as you grow older, you may become more doubtful and even skeptical, and you might even have ceased to have confidence in yourself anymore. But to regain your self-confidence, you must set goals, and achieve as many of them as possible.

The only stumbling block is your inability to achieve some of your goals at some points in your life. This may then create negativity in the form of *victimization*. That is to say, you may erroneously believe that you are a victim of circumstances; this self-delusion may also lead to anger, bitterness, despair, and many other negative emotions that debilitate you in reaching your life goals. The end result: you feel depressed.

> "Without awe of the mysteries of the Creator,
> we are easily controlled by fear.
> Without self-love and compassion for others,
> we are easily victimized by others."
> (Lao Tzu, *Tao Te Ching*, Chapter 72)

## TAO wisdom

Setting goals and having expectations are not the same. According to TAO, expectations often come with a price. The greater your expectations, the more efforts you will want to exert, and the more stressed you may become— ironically enough, that may lead to failure in achieving your goals. TAO recommends "doing what needs to be done" but no more and no less, and with "no expectation" of the outcome of all your efforts. In other words, setting and working at life goals focuses only on the process, and not on the outcome, which is one of the essentials of TAO.

> "We are all desirous of making the right choices,
> fearful of making the wrong ones.
> We all pursue what others say is good,
> avoiding what they say is bad.
> We all follow the popular wisdom of judgment

and preference,
instead of the wisdom of the Creator,
requiring us to be undesirous and unperturbed,
just like a newborn."
(Lao Tzu, **Tao Te Ching**, Chapter 20)

Being unable to accomplish your life goals may further make you start comparing and contrasting yourself with others, and thus emphasizing your own inadequacy and shortcomings. TAO says you should never compare and contrast with others; instead, seeing the oneness of all life may help you understand that we all have our own shortcomings and weaknesses, and that nobody is perfect in achieving all his or her life goals.

"Knowing our true nature,
we know who we are,
and what we need.
We accomplish things
without taking credit or reward.
We cherish ourselves
without separating us from other beings.
We nourish our external identity
without forgetting our inner reality."
(Lao Tzu, *Tao Te Ching*, Chapter 72)

Self-confidence, together with the TAO of "no over-doing" and "no expectation," holds the key to setting your life goals and accomplishing as many of them as possible, but without being held back by any drawback and difficulty encountered along the way. Gradually and consistently building up your self-confidence is necessary for success in doing anything in your life.

Always remember this ultimate TAO reality:

"The ultimate truths have to be self-intuited:
be simple, be selfless, and be non-judgmental.
Enlightenment may arrive effortlessly."
(Lao Tzu, *Tao Te Ching*, Chapter 19)

Always live your life on your own terms without any fear of rejection or disappointment. Always accept and embrace everything as you seek your life goals.

## (10) Health and Wisdom

Happiness and good health go hand-in-hand. Indeed, scientific studies have found that happiness can give you a healthier heart, a much stronger immune system, and even a longer lifespan with less stress.

Wisdom is essential to staying healthy as you continue to plod along your life journey, especially if you are heading towards your final destination.

### Biblical Wisdom

Generally, many so-called believers often pray to their God for three things: be happy, be healthy, and be wealthy. There is no rhyme or reason for these prayers: if one is depressed, how can one be happy, even if one is wealthy?

## *Health attitudes*

To be healthy, that is, at least free from depression, an individual may have different health attitudes. In general, people express different attitudes towards their own health:

### Attitude of despair

Those, who have been plagued by ill health, need faith to rejuvenate their love of health.

Despair is a sin against God. According to **C.S. Lewis**, "despair is greater than any of the sins that provoke it."

### Attitude of confusion

Those, who do not know *how* to pursue good health, need faith to illuminate their love of health.

God will shed light and show you the way all for the asking.

> Ask, and it will be given to you; seek, and you will find; knock, and it will be opened to you. (**Matthew** 7:7)

### Attitude of complacency

Those, who have been enjoying relatively good health, need faith to enhance, if not to sustain or rediscover, their love of health.

## *Love of health*

It is not enough just to avoid doing wrong: God wants you to be *proactive* about doing what is *right* for your health.

Health is man's greatest asset. Therefore, you should express your love of health. If your love of health is like your faith in your search for God, you will have your reward. It all begins with *love*—the love of God, the love of life, which is a gift from Him, and hence the love of health.

He who pursues righteousness and loyalty finds
life, righteousness, and honor.
(**Proverbs** 21:21)

Love of health is more than just a desire for physical
health, which is contingent on spiritual and mental wellness
as well.

Life is a sacred journey involving change, growth, and
self-discovery. Knowledge is empowering. Therefore, for
your love of heath, you should seek knowledge continually
to expand your vision and stretch your soul in order to stay
spiritually, physically, and mentally healthy. Your spirituality
provides meaning and direction, which is wisdom, for the
body on that life journey. With wisdom, you may become
enlightened. You will realize that natural health holds the
key to your overall well-being.

The Bible says that God's "people are destroyed for lack
of knowledge." (**Hosea** 4:6) Do not destroy your love of
health for lack of knowledge and wisdom.

For someone who is very ill, it may seem difficult,
almost impossible, to restore natural health and to get well
again. Worse, ill health may make you forget to take care of
your body, and thus allowing your body's functions to
deteriorate further. But if you are living with spiritual
wisdom, all things are possible.

To regain natural health, you need a vision of good
health and wholeness. You must always attune yourself to
Nature's natural laws of balance and harmony, expressed
by your body's inner healing intelligence, which allows your
body to repair and heal itself.

Ill health is no more than the accumulation of all the
wrong things you have done to your body over the years.
For the love of health, stop poisoning your body with

processed foods and pharmaceutical drugs. For the love of health, eat healthy, and stop your toxic food cravings. Always use food as your medicine.

> Then God said, 'Behold, I have given you every plant yielding seed that is on the surface of all the earth, and every tree which has fruit yielding seed; it shall be food for you;
> (**Genesis** 1:29)

You have to make your food choices each and every day of your life—food choices that are life-enhancing or death-inducing. The choice is all yours. Living in faith, you will find it much easier to make healthful choices in your lifestyle, such as giving up your addiction to alcohol and nicotine. You have to make a decision to involve your Creator in your everyday living in order to provide you with strength and wisdom to overcome your daily challenge in matters of food choices.

> I can do all things through Him who strengthens me.
> (**Philippians** 4:13)

> that He would grant you, according to the riches of His glory, to be strengthened with power through His spirit in the inner man,
> (**Ephesians** 3:16)

To sustain rejuvenation and recovery, it is important to detoxify your body regularly through fasting, natural herbs, such as dandelion, licorice, and milk thistle, and vegetables, such as beets and broccoli.

Then Jesus was led up by the Spirit into the
wilderness to be tempted by the devil. And
after He had fasted forty days and forty nights,
He then became hungry.
(**Matthew** 4:1-2)

**Jesus** demonstrates that fasting can purify the mind and
the body. In addition, He shows that without faith, it is
easier to relapse into bad eating habits and unhealthful
lifestyle.

Do you not know that you are a temple of God
and that the Spirit of God dwells in you? If any
man destroys the temple of God, God will
destroy him, for the temple of God is holy, and
this is what you are.
(**I Corinthians** 3:16-17)

## Living in faith

Your body is the temple of the Holy Spirit. Therefore,
treat your body with respect so that it may last a longer
time.

Living in faith is a tall order in life. Believe that **Jesus**
came into this world that you may "have life and have it
abundantly." (**John** 10:10) as well as "prosper and be in
good health, just as your soul prospers." (**3 John**: 2)

God does not want you to be in bondage to fad diets,
overeating, or harmful substances. Instead, He wants you
to be free and to exercise self-control in all areas of your
life, including your food choices, through living in spiritual
wisdom. Always use food as your medicine, and not as a
distraction from your depression.

If you do not take care of your body, and yet you expect

God to fix your physical ailments right away—that is *not* spiritual wisdom!

Spiritual wisdom is to believe that God will do His best to take care of your body, *if* you will also do your best to take care of His creation by eating right.

The bottom line is the axiom: you reap what you sow, and you become what you eat.

> But you shall serve the Lord your God, and He will bless your bread and water; and I will remove sickness from your midst.
> (**Exodus** 23:5)

So, do not pray for "be happy" or "be wealthy," but for the spiritual wisdom to "be healthy."

## Spiritual Wisdom

Even if you are a non-Christian, or a believer in other faith, you may also have spiritual wisdom. Not to mention the atheists, most people still believe in the existence of a Higher Being, who is in control of many inexplicable things in the universe, such as the presence of the sun.

The truth of the matter is that spirituality may still be present in the hearts of many because they still believe that they all have a soul, which is essentially an unfathomable human spirit. As opposed to materiality, spirituality is always invisible, immeasurable, but forever present and lasting. Like the wind, invisible and yet palpable, it may provide the mind or the soul of an individual with direction, guidance, and understanding. Spirituality may take the form of love, joy, and peace, and it is often expressed in human actions and behaviors. Materiality, on the other hand, is always visible, measurable, and transient.

Humans need *both* spirituality and materiality: the former to understand self, and the latter to understand the world and the universe around the self. Spirituality not only inspires the mind but also energizes the body—it is an intricate and inexplicable body-mind connection that is essential to the art of living well in the material world.

Use *awareness* to enhance your inherent spirituality: be aware of your body-mind-soul connection. Living in the physical world is challenging in itself. The many challenges often turn themselves into toxins that contaminate the body as well as the mind. A mind is supposed to control the body, but a festered mind loses much of its control over the body, and thus letting the body poison not only itself but also the mind as well. Spiritual wisdom may be able to provide the mind with instructions and inspirations on *how* to take care of the body, such as a change of diet and lifestyle.

## TAO wisdom

TAO says you should not label yourself sick. Sickness is not a normal human condition. Labeling only compounds the problem of sickness, because we are already living in a world of depression, and the whole world is medicine. What is the sickness? Maybe, only the sickness of the mind.

According to TAO, live your life fully and actively, that is, experiencing *everything* you come across in your life, including your depression.

Eat a balanced, varied, and healthful diet. Choosing a *specific* diet never works, because you need to shift your diet to accommodate to the ever-changing needs of your body. Accordingly, you have to *listen* to your body. No food is a perfect balance.

Exercise plays a pivotal part in health and wellness.

Exercise, however, has to demonstrate a moderate level of effort.

Lead a stress-free life, instead of making your life a continuous fight and struggle against others and the world; excess resistance not only wears you down but also erodes your eternal energy for balance and harmony, which is the essence of good health.

> "In natural harmony with the Creator,
> we let all things come and go,
> exerting no effort, showing no desire,
> and expecting no result.
> Natural harmony is experienced
> only in the present moment,
> when we see the natural laws of the Creator."
> (Lao Tzu, *Tao Te Ching*, Chapter 55)

Live as who you are. Avoid all addictions, which erase and erode your unique nature, and lead to a dead end in the pathway of your life. Addictions may include, addiction to alcohol, drugs, medications, and even to the media.

Once you begin putting TAO into practice, your health will begin to improve, your mind will slowly get clearer, and new solutions to your health problems may even appear for you to take step-by-step towards recovery and rejuvenation.

> "We neither strain nor stress.
> We let go of success and failure.
> We patiently take the next necessary step,
> a small step and one step at a time.
> We relinquish our conditioned thinking.
> Being our true nature, we help all beings
> return to their own true nature too."
> (Lao Tzu, *Tao Te Ching*, Chapter 64)

The truth of putting TAO into practice is that you just have to be open to acceptance: accepting that you are indeed complete and wholesome, which in fact we all are, every moment of your life.

> "It is hidden, but forever present.
> It is inconceivable and intangible.
> It comes from the Creator, the origin of all things."
> (Lao Tzu, *Tao Te Ching*, Chapter 4)

## (11) Changes and Challenges

Life is forever changing. A static life is not worth living. Ironically enough, many people resist any change in their lives; they desire consistency and stability. Unfortunately, whether you like it or not, changes are inevitable as you continue to age. The Way is the only way to cope with life changes: adaptability and acceptance.

## Adaptability and Acceptance

Adaptability is changing the mind's perception of the changes you confront, and act or react accordingly to the circumstances. This mental perception requires *awareness*, without which actions or reactions may not even take place, because often times changes are slow, gradual, and even subtly imperceptible to the human mind. Awareness means knowing *why* and *how* changes are taking place.

> "We need a still and composed mind
> to see things with greater clarity.
> Because trouble begins in the mind

with small and unrelated thoughts.
So, we carefully watch the mind
to stop any trouble before it begins."
(Lao Tzu, *Tao Te Ching*, Chapter 64)

Acceptance is taking the responsibility of the results of the actions or reactions taken. Acceptance may not be easy, especially if you already have a conditioned mindset of expectation, or that of comparing the conditions before and after the change.

Both adaptability and acceptance requires *wisdom*—the wisdom to know and understand that nothing is permanent because everything remains only with that very present moment, and that everything follows the natural cycle, such as success as followed by failure.

"Success and failure are no more than expressions of the human condition.
So, accept both gracefully and willingly, with no judgment, no preference.
The Creator loves us unconditionally, irrespective of our success or failure.
What is meant by 'accept both gracefully and willingly'?
Success is avoiding failure; avoiding failure is seeking success.
Both originate from fear and pride: the sources of human suffering.
Seeing ourselves indiscriminately as everything, including success and failure,
we see not only the manifestations but also the mysteries of the creation."
(Lao Tzu, *Tao Te Ching*, Chapter 13)

Adaptability gives flexibility, which is internal vitality, essential to life and living.

"At birth, we are soft and supple.
At death, we are stiff and hard.
Young plants are tender and pliant.
Dead plants are brittle and dry.

Stiff and inflexible, we are like death.
Soft and yielding, we are like life.

Following the Way,
we become soft and supple.
That is why we always prevail,
because tenderness and flexibility
give us strength and power from the Creator."
(Lao Tzu, *Tao Te Ching*, Chapter 76)

## Letting Go

On August 26, 2015, **Vester Flanagan** gunned down CBS reporter **Alison Parker** and photojournalist **Adam Ward** in front of the TV camera; this vicious slaughter was witnessed by thousands of TV viewers in the United States. The shooter was a former reporter of a CBS-affiliated television station, and he was fired in 2013 due to his disruptive misbehavior.

Many TV viewers of that cold-blooded slaughter, including some of the interviewed psychologists, tried to explain *why* the murderer would do such a horrific act.

Maybe the gunman had a mind disorder. Maybe the mind disorder was a result of not "letting go" of his former animosity workplace.

In life, we all have to learn how to let go of *everything*, including life itself, when we have to confront imminent death as a result of ill health or old age. Throughout life, we have to let go of our children when they go to college, get married, or sometimes even die ahead of us; we have to let go of material things, such as career, money, and so on and so forth; we have to let go of our memories—memories of the unpleasant in the form of anger, bitterness, or vengeance, as well as memories of the pleasant in the form of desires and expectations. If we do not and cannot let go of our emotions, we may develop a mind disorder, which is depression.

This is *how* the mind disorder of a killer, such as Vester Flanagan, is developed. An individual is fired from his job. That individual's own perceptions of disappointment, discrimination, dissatisfaction, injustice, racial prejudice, and among many others, become registered in the mind as memories. Without the power of letting go of these mind-devastating memories, that individual will continue to generate many more negative thoughts in the subconscious mind until the breaking point. If that individual has an aggressive or a violent nature, then killing may seem to be the unavoidable last resort, and the only way out of that depressive mind disorder.

It is all about letting go, which is one of the essentials of TAO. To learn how to let go, begin with your letting go of material things. Are you living a simple life? Is your closet cluttered with clothes that you have not worn in the past few years? Then, learn to let go of time. Are you always on the go? Do you do texting while driving? Are you living in the past or the future, except in the present? Finally, let go of your memories Do you easily forgive or do you always bear grudges? If you do not let go, you may have anger, anxiety, and other mind disorders, including depression, that may even culminate in tragedies.

"Letting go is emptying the mundane,
to be filled with heavenly grace.

Blessed is he who has an empty mind.
He will be filled with knowledge and wisdom from the Creator.
Blessed is he who has no attachment to worldly things.
He will be compensated with heavenly riches."
(Lao Tzu, *Tao Te Ching*, Chapter 9)

## TAO wisdom

The reality, whether we like it or not, is that everything in this world is impermanent because everything is forever changing. So, why do you fight a battle that has no chance of winning? Just be an observer of the combats of others, instead of becoming a participant yourself.

"The Creator seems elusive amid the changes of life.
At times, He seems to have forsaken His creations.
In reality, He is simply observing the comings and goings of their follies.

Likewise, we watch the comings and goings of our likes and dislikes, of our desires and fears.
But we do not identify with them.
With no judgment and no preference,

we see the mysteries of creation."
(Lao Tzu, *Tao Te Ching*, Chapter 7)

TAO is the only way *through* anything and everything in life.

> "Can we embrace both good fortunes and misfortunes in life?
> Can we breathe as easily as innocent babies?
> Can we see the world created as is without judgment?
> Can we accept both the desirable and the undesirable?
> Can we express compassion to all without being boastful?
> Can we watch the comings and goings of things without being perturbed?
> Saying "yes" to all of the above is spiritual wisdom from the Creator,
> who watches the comings and goings in the world He created."
> (Lao Tzu, *Tao Te Ching*, Chapter 10)

Just follow TAO *through* your depression.

## (12) Death and Adversity

Life is never smooth sailing, and life journey is forever a bumpy ride. No matter how you look at your life or that of someone else, even if it may look like a bed of roses, it always has some thorns. Death and adversity always appear on the roadsides along your life journey.

## Fear of Death

If you have lived long enough, or being aware that you are approaching the destination of your life journey, you may become obsessed with the fear of death, which is no more than the consciousness of the unknown ahead. That explains why many seniors become depressed.

TAO wisdom

According to TAO, death is a natural destination of the Way—going back to its origin.

> "Abiding in the Creator, we do not fear death.
> Following the conditioned mind, we fear everything.
> Fear is a futile attempt to control things and people.
>
> Death is a natural destination of the Way.
> Unnatural fear of death does more harm than good.
> It is like trying to use intricate tools of a master craftsman:
> we end up hurting ourselves."
> (Lao Tzu, *Tao Te Ching*, Chapter 74)

So, you should neither ignore death nor be obsessed with it; just live your life as if there is no tomorrow, while experiencing *everything* to the fullest.

> "Life begets death; one is inseparable from the other.
> One is form; the other is formless.
> Each gives way to the other.

One third of people focus on life, ignoring death.
One third of people focus on death, ignoring life.
One third of people think of neither, just drifting along.
They all suffer in the end.

Trusting the Creator, we have no illusion about life and death.
Holding nothing back from life, we are ready for death,
just as a man ready for sleep after a good day's work."

(Lao Tzu, *Tao Te Ching*, Chapter 50)

## Sorrow and Suffering

Emotional pain and suffering due to death and bereavement often become the bag and baggage that many seniors carry with them until they reach the destinations of their life journeys.

After the death of a dear friend or someone close to you, you may experience a period of *denial*—refusing to accept the harsh reality of death. This is the human mind's natural way of *escape* from the painful emotions associated with grief and sorrow.

Sorrow and suffering may then bring *anger*: anger with yourself or whoever responsible for the death of your loved one. The human mind always looks for an answer or an explanation of *why* something undesirable has happened. If you blame yourself, then guilt and regret may ensue; if you blame others, anger is generated. According to TAO, anger is the source of human sufferings. Anger originates from desires and expectations that are not met or fulfilled.

The next phase is *bargaining* with God about reversing what happened to you. You may even use pleas, such as "what if?" and "if only" to bargain for your second chances, as demonstrated by **Jesus'** own pleading: "My Father, if it is possible, let this cup pass from Me." (**Matthew** 26:39)

After the initial denial and bargaining, reality begins to sink in. You may start to feel the bereavement that causes you to sink into deep depression with negative emotions of grief, regret, and sorrow. This is the darkest or even the longest phase of grief and sorrow.

TAO wisdom

TAO emphasizes the dualism of life: that is, good and bad co-exist, just as happiness and sorrow, and they complement each other. Without sorrow, there will be no happiness, and one gives way to the other somehow and some time.

"Likewise, life and death complement each other.
Heaven is eternal life; hell is everlasting death.
Human existence is therefore dualistic:
it can make heaven out of hell, or hell out of heaven."
(Lao Tzu, *Tao Te Ching*, Chapter 2)

TAO says you should live in the present, and not the past which was gone, or the future which is yet to come. According to TAO, you simply embrace whatever that comes along in your life without any judgment.

*Spontaneity* is of one the essentials of TAO; it means everything in life follows a certain natural and spontaneous order, such as the four seasons, or life becoming death. Understanding the natural order of all things may deliver you from your depression and lift you out of the darkness of pain and sorrow.

The only way to overcome pain and sorrow is *acceptance*. Sooner or later, you will come to terms with the death of your loved one when you become aware that everything is going to be okay, that you will survive the loss of your loved one, and go on living as if everything is a miracle even though your life may be quite different without your loved one.

Given that everything is this world is *impermanent*, grief and sorrow are also impermanent. So, do not let your grief and sorrow make you unhappy over the long haul; protracted grief and sorrow may lead to deeper depression and more negative thoughts that may haunt you for the rest of your life.

Overcoming grief and sorrow requires you to process your grief and sorrow with TAO by experiencing and living *through* every aspect of your grief and sorrow before there is any healing or redemption from any emotional pain and suffering. You must let your sorrow and suffering run their natural courses until you can express and share them with others to complement the healing process.

Above all, your healing and redemption demand an honest understanding of *who* you really are, and *why* you are here in this material world; in other words, your connection or re-connection with your Creator. TAO suggests you to look inward, and not outward.

> "We always look for the visible and the tangible without.

But what really matters is the invisible and the intangible within."
(Lao Tzu, *Tao Te Ching*, Chapter 11)

Therefore, it is important that as a Christian or a believer of faith in God, you have to die to self—that is, you have to give up your comfort zone, and experience the realm of emotional pain, just as **Jesus** did: "My Father, if this cannot pass away unless I drink it, Your will be done." (**Matthew** 26:42)

**Jesus** wanted us to follow His example too. *That* is the spiritual wisdom that He wants to give us.

We will all experience loss, hurt, and rejection in our lives at one time or another—it is the reality that we must all face, and living in faith is the only way to confront this reality. Remember, instant peace only leads to recurrent emotional pain because there is no real healing from painful emotions without the faith to die to self to fully embrace sorrow and suffering just as **Jesus** did. This is similar to TAO's letting-go: we all come from nothing and will, therefore, return to nothing. But nothingness is in fact *everything*.

"We watch everything come and go,
with no judgment, no preference.
Everything that is, was, or ever will be,
will return to its origin: the Creator.

Understanding the comings and goings of things,
we fret not, and judge not."
(Lao Tzu, *Tao Te Ching*, Chapter 16)

To enhance this spiritual wisdom of TAO, you must

lead a simple life, letting go of all attachments in your bag and baggage.

> "The more we look, the less we see.
> The more we hear, the less we listen.
> The more we crave, the crazier we become.
>
> What is materialistic is separate from what is spiritualistic.
> Therefore, value what is within, and not what is without."
> (Lao Tzu, *Tao Te Ching*, Chapter 12)

## Adversity and Pain

Adversity is also part and parcel of life and living. Adversity coming in different phases in life only becomes more challenging and noticeable in your advanced years. Therefore, it is important to understand the nature of adversity in order to cope with it, and not necessarily to overcome it.

Adversity is like the rites of passage, which come in three stages: the separation stage in which you feel separated from your comfort zone; the confusion stage in which you find yourself in no-man's-land, at a complete loss of not knowing what to do next; and then the transformation stage, in which you initiate your changes to cope with the adversity.

Pain, due to adversity, may come in different forms: emotional, physical, mental, and spiritual pain. Inevitable as it is, pain also comes in different stages of life, and most predominantly during the last years as a result of loss of loved ones, loss of physical capability and functioning, as well as loss of health and wellness.

According to **Dr. Albert Schweitzer**, "Pain is a more terrible lord of mankind than even death itself, and awakens us to a courage and faith unrealized before."

No matter what, your last years will ultimately dwindle into your last days of peace and harmony—what is experienced by those who have accepted and embraced pain. Humor and laughter are the only antidotes to pain.

**Norman Cousins**, in his book *Anatomy of an Illness*, was able to cure himself of his terminal cancer by exposing himself to as much humor as he could get from movies and comic books. No matter what, smile, laugh, and develop a good sense of humor.

## Smiling

Babies begin smiling within the first few weeks of life, and laugh out loud within months of being born because laughter is a natural, positive response to human life. Sadly, as human life progresses, laughter may even begin to fade away into oblivion.

But laughter is especially important to you in the last chapters of your life because it overcomes adversities and all bad feelings about yourself, others, or what is happening to you. Laughter is your best medicine in your last days: it releases endorphins to make you feel good about yourself no matter what; it protects your heart by improving blood flow to your heart; it reduces your stress hormones, thereby boosting your immune system; it relaxes your body and mind to enable you to enjoy living in the present; it makes you forget your lingering physical and emotional pain. Laughter is your natural medicine for you as you approach the final destination of your life journey.

## Humor

While laughter is instantaneous, humor is always subtle, gradual, but infectious. The major role of humor in life is to change your perspectives of what is happening to you. It enables you to look at yourself in a less serious manner. Since you are approaching the end of your life journey, why should you look upon life so seriously? Weave humor into the fabrics of your life: let yourself find good humor in almost everything you do. Remind yourself that you are much more blessed than most people—for one thing, you already have lived to a ripe old age—and that many things are beyond your control anyway, so loosen up your tight jaw and start smiling. Laugh at yourself by sharing some embarrassing moments in your life with those who are also fun and playful. Look for humor in any bad situation; if you look further, you will always find the irony and absurdity of life. Above all, make a conscious effort to overcome your daily stress, which is a major impediment to laughter and humor.

According to the 2006 *International Journal of Psychiatry in Medicine*, a sense of humor can significantly improve the survival rate of end-stage renal disease patients by as much as 30 percent. The reason is simple: positive distractions from stressful situations, such as dialysis, have salutary effects on the patient.

Remember, if you just continue to live, you will also continue to face many adversities. Laughter and humor will let you see only their positive sides, instead of becoming the problem yourself.

You do not have to be funny in order to have a sense of humor—just the ability to see the lighter side of everything in life. Now that you are nearing the end of your life journey, nothing can be that dead serious—not even death.

*Developing a sense of humor*

Developing your sense of humor requires a different perspective on all things in life. Changing your perspective means going back through your entire life and looking at all the belief systems that you have inculcated through different experiences in different stages of your life. It is not as simple as you may think, but it is worth the effort, because a good sense of humor may help you in your adversity Life is full of problems, especially in the last golden days. A good sense of humor controls how you *see* your problems in your daily life.

TAO wisdom

TAO may help you develop a good sense of humor.

Always see yourself not in the center of things, but rather a part of it. Your problems may not be uniquely yours; others, too, may have the same problems, or even worse than yours for that matter. Do not be too self-centered that you are always bearing the blunt.

Never take yourself too seriously. Just learn to laugh at yourself—your mistakes, your foolishness, and even your weaknesses. Remember, nobody is perfect!

> "Life lives itself in us, when we focus on the Creator.
> From that focal point, around which all of life revolves."
> (Lao Tzu, *Tao Te Ching*, Chapter 16)

Live in the present. Everything is constantly changing, including your body and thoughts. Everything in life can only be experienced in each moment, and moment by moment, which is the only reality. Live in the present moment, appreciate it, and enjoy it to the fullest. When you do just that, you may see not only the humor but also the absurdity of everything around you, especially in the past.

Always putting a smile on your face not only helps you develop a sense of humor but also gives joy to others. Remember, a smile is contagious. There is no harm in smiling—even in any bad situation.

Make a list of all the things you enjoy in life—things that really make you happy. Remember and recall them at all times.

If you can *laugh* at yourself and join in with the laughter of others, it can bring not only much more joy but also many more golden days to your life.

## (13) Unfairness and Inequality

One of the main triggers of human depression is a feeling of unfairness and inequality that may stem from our perceptions and comparisons with others. This trigger raises many internal questions that we often ask when we are alone by ourselves: "I am smarter than my brother, but why is it that he is having a better destiny than mine?"; "My daughter is the prettiest among all her friends, but why is it that she doesn't even have a boyfriend?"; "My father is a very nice person, but why is it that everyone is taking advantage of him?"; "My former neighbor stole money from the company he used to work with, and now he is the CEO of this big corporate company, where is the justice?"

Don't we all have many similar questions unanswered? If we continue to look for answers to those unanswerable questions, we would only succumb ourselves to depression. In life, there are many questions that we may never have an answer simply because of the following:

- We are limited in our knowledge, and we always see only one side of everything.
- Our perceptions are inaccurate because we all have too many implicit assumptions.
- We are finite: we see only the present and, at most, the nearest future. The Creator is infinite, and to Him everything is timeless and happens only according to His timetable.

But many of us still demand some sort of answers to satisfy our desire for fairness and equality, not to mention justice. In life, there are many questions which may never have an answer. But in TAO, the answer is always deep within us.

## A case in point

In 1984, **Archbishop Valerian Trifa** was deported from the United States after being accused of being a Nazi supporter, who had incited attacks on Jews, and was responsible for executing many civilians in World War II.

After World War II, the Nazi supporter came to the United States as a refugee immigrant. He assumed the name of Valerian Trifa, and was ordained as a priest of the Rumanian church soon after his arrival in the United States. He rose quickly to the rank of bishop and archbishop, and lived in comfort in a 25-room farmhouse on a 200-acre estate maintained by his church.

Later on, a dentist, who was a Nazi survivor, recognized the Archbishop as the Nazi supporter. The case against him was then pursued for more than a decade by survivors of the Nazi years, Jewish organizations, journalists, and the

Justice Department of the United States. Their efforts helped focus public attention on Nazi war criminals who were living in the United States.

At first, the Archbishop vehemently denied his former identity, despite some handwriting experts confirming that his handwriting was identical with that in some of the execution orders he had carried out while he was a Nazi supporter. As luck would have it, with the advancement of forensic science, some experts could incredibly still retrieve some DNA from those execution orders. That was his undoing, and his final judgment.

The Archbishop was ultimately ordered to leave the United States in 1982, but spent two years trying to find a country that would give him refuge. Portugal admitted him in 1984, and he finally settled in Estoril, where he died of a heart attack at the age of 72.

The reality

Archbishop Valerian Trifa had undergone decades of denial and prosecution. Nobody knows what was going on in his mind while he was the Archbishop and during those years of prosecution. The reality is that he thought he could get away with murder, but the past came back to haunt him.

TAO wisdom

TAO teaches that the Creator is in absolute control of everything that happens in this world, but only according to His own timetable. His "vast net" is all-encompassing and all-inclusive, and nothing slips through it.

"We try to be good, and do the best we can,

yet sometimes bad things happen to us.
We have no explanation for that.
We just follow the Way,
one step at a time,
accepting the good and the bad,
as essential parts of life.
We quietly respond to every situation
with neither strain nor stress.

We trust the Creator.
His net, vast and loose,
covers the whole universe,
and nothing slips through.
He controls all."
(Lao Tzu, *Tao Te Ching*, Chapter 73)

"When we are separate from our true nature,
we experience no natural goodness,
no compassion and no loving-kindness.
Our goodness then becomes contrived,
demanding fairness and justice,
focusing on appearance and superficiality."
(Lao Tzu, *Tao Te Ching*, Chapter 38)

The bottom line, do not waste your internal energy by striving to seek answers to those unanswered questions about unfairness, inequality, or injustice. Just accept and embrace whatever happens in your life, and the Creator will take care of i. Just leave everything to Him.

Do not fret because of those who are evil
    or be envious of those who do wrong;
for like the grass they will soon wither,
    like green plants they will soon die away.

Trust in the LORD and do good;
    dwell in the land and enjoy safe pasture.
Take delight in the LORD,
    and he will give you the desires of your
heart.
(**Psalm** 37: 1-4)

## (14) The Conclusion

There is no way out of depression, except *through* TAO, which is the Way.

All paths are aspects of the one path, just as all truths are aspects of the one truth, which is TAO.

To follow the pathless path to TAO, you must have the empty and inquisitive mindset of a child, who is ready and willing to explore and to experience anything and every-thing that may come along.

Children are considered a gift from God because they care for their older parents and carry on the family name when their parents die. Yet children have little power and have to obey their parents completely. Even **Jesus** used children as an example to show that being powerful is not the way to get into God's kingdom; what God really wants is only our *trust* and *obedience*.

> Let the little children come to me, and do not
> hinder them, for the kingdom of God belongs
> to such as these.
> (**Mark** 10: 14)

Likewise, TAO focuses on obeying and observing the laws of Nature without any resistance in order to attain internal balance and harmony to live and survive in this world of depression.

In the spiritual world, your Creator will not judge you for your success or failure, but He will judge you for not being who you were created for and meant to be. Your most important obligation in this world is to be your true self to live the life you are meant to live. Never ever compare yourself with others, or wish you were someone else!

Being your true self without an inflated ego is humility which is the essence of TAO. Likewise, human humility is always pleasing to God, and will be rewarded with spiritual wisdom. With humility, you become aligned with the Creator, who provides us with the wisdom to live in this material world.

Living in this material world, we all strive to create an identity for ourselves, we all want to be different from others, and that is why we all have a name. An ego-self is the beginning of pride, which is the first of the Seven Deadly Sins, and the cause of the fall of man. With an ego-self, we begin to set goals in our lives to define our identities, to distinguish us from others. Once the goals are set, we expect to meet all of them, as well as to meet the expectations from others around us. With expectations, we tend to judge, which means picking and choosing what we want and rejecting what we do not want; we begin to like and dislike, because we want to accomplish our goals that will satisfy our ego-self. Throughout this process of judgment, we no longer live in the present moment, because our minds are preoccupied with thoughts of repeating our success in the past and avoiding our failure in the future. Not only are we not living in the present, we are "over-doing" everything in order to get what we want to satisfy the pride of the ego-self.

The once-celebrated-and-now-dishonored cyclist **Lance Armstrong** best illustrates all the components of TAO.

He was once a celebrated Olympic cyclist decorated with most medals and honors, but was stripped of everything when he was caught doping with performance-enhancing drugs.

You want to be the best cyclist in the world (ego-self). You expect yourself to work hard to meet the expectations of others, including yourself (expectations). You begin to choose what is best to achieve your goals, including doping (picking and choosing based on judgment). You are no longer concerned about your health or the legal issues of doping (not living in the present). You over-do everything, including excessive practice, doping, and manipulating other cyclists (over-doing). Think about all your striving, straining, and strutting just for the sake of satisfying your ego-self! But also think about the price you may have to pay for that!

Humility is always within our reach because it is inherent in human nature, just as **Ann Frank** in "The Diary of Ann Frank" said, "Human worth does not lie in riches or power, but in character or goodness."

Having said that, to fully understand and appreciate the pivotal role of humility in everyday life and living, especially with respect to depression, may not be easy for many of us, given that we all have an ego-self to deal with. Therefore, spiritual wisdom is necessary to provide the guidance and inspiration, and TAO is the Way to that wisdom.

"The Creator is above,
and we are below.
The Creator is in front,
and we are behind.
Because this is the nature of things,
humility is only natural to us.
Yet many are desirous of the top

fearful of lagging behind.
Humility is the Way."
(Lao Tzu, *Tao Te Ching*, Chapter 66)

With humility, finding the Way is easy.

"The Way is easy to find and follow:
empty the mind of conditioned thinking
of seeing things and doing things.

The Way comes from the source of all.
Its power cherishes and nourishes all.
Knowing the source, we know ourselves.

Finding the Way,
we know the nature of things;
we see the comings and goings of things.

Following the Way,
we discover the treasures within;
we simplify the trappings without.
So, we continue the Way with inner joy."
(Lao Tzu, *Tao Te Ching*, Chapter 70)

Go *through* your depression with TAO to experience *everything* in life, instead of avoiding all the unhappy as well as the unpleasant, and you may become enlightened.

# APPENDIX A

## A SUMMARY OF TAO WISDOM

The eternal wisdom of TAO can be summarized in the following self-intuitive questions and answers:

**Who am I?**

You are not *who* you think you really are.

**Why is that?**

Your mind tells you who you are—not what you or others say you have done

**Then, why is it that I am not who I am if my mind says so?**

Your mind is deceiving you, or you unconsciously let your mind deceive yourself.

**Do I create my own delusion and self-deception?**

You do not *consciously* create your own delusion and self-deception, but *subconsciously* you do.

**How do I do that?**

You create your thoughts through your thinking mind, not your knowledge mind. Your thoughts are stored in your subconscious mind, which also projects them as future thoughts into your subconscious mind. They become *your* thoughts, and they *seem* real to you, but, in fact, they are not. It is like you are standing in front of a mirror. It seems that there are two persons there. But the one in the mirror is only a reflection, and is intangible and non-existent.

**Why do I create these thoughts if they are not real?**

It is because you crave an identity, and your mind tells you to identify yourself with these thoughts, both past and future, to create your ego-self.

**How do I stop my mind from creating these "unreal" thoughts?**

By staying in the present moment, which is the only reality: the past was gone and the future is uncertain and unpredictable.

**How do I stay in the present moment?**

Focus on something insignificant or irrelevant, such as breathing. When you are in the present moment, you become an observer of your past and future thoughts, and you are no longer an active participant. As such, you can see who you really are, or observe your ego-self more objectively without any judgment.

**Do I have an ego-self?**

Yes, you do, just like everyone else. Just learn to let go of your ego-self, as much as possible.

### What happens when I have no ego-self?

Then you may have a better understanding of TAO wisdom.

### How do I become enlightened?

You become enlightened only when you have full real-life applications of TAO.

### What happens when I let go of my ego-self?

You become just a being, observing what is happening to that being; you begin to lose your attachments, your cravings, your expectations. You begin to live your life as it is, accepting and embracing everything, instead of resisting and denying its very existence. That is, you live as if everything is a miracle.

### When can one become enlightened?

When one has the answer to every question in life—or when one stops asking any more questions because one already has all the answers, which are in TAO.

Remember, wisdom is like a plant. Cultivate it, and watch it grow, and it will blossom. Just be present as the observer of your mind, of your thoughts, of your emotions and feelings, as well as of your actions and reactions to them.

TAO is all transformative: transforming apathy into

empathy, harm into harmony, meaningless existence into meaningful life, and potentials into realities.

With TAO, you may still have your depression, but you simply experience it quite *differently*.

"The truth is unpleasant to the ear.
What is pleasant to the ear is not the truth.
Likewise, true wisdom is unpopular;
what is popular is not true wisdom."
(Lao Tzu, *Tao Te Ching*, Chapter 81)

"The Way is easy to find and follow:
empty the mind of conditioned thinking
of seeing things and doing things.

The Way comes from the source of all.
Its power cherishes and nourishes all.
Knowing the source, we know ourselves.

Finding the Way,
we know the nature of things;
we see the comings and goings of things.

Following the Way,
we discover the treasures within;
we simplify the trappings without.
So, we continue the Way with inner joy."
(Lao Tzu, *Tao Te Ching*, Chapter 70)

# APPENDIX B

# DIAPHRAGM BREATHING

Always use your diaphragm (the diaphragm muscle separating your chest from your abdomen) to breathe, and not your lungs. Essentially, when your diaphragm goes down, you lungs fill up with air; when your diaphragm goes up, your lungs push the air out, expelling the toxic carbon dioxide. Incomplete breathing (when you use your lungs, instead of the diaphragm, to breathe in and breathe out) leads to accumulation of toxic wastes in the lungs and in other parts of your body organs and tissues. Diaphragm breathing is correct breathing to boost health and wellness of both the body and the mind.

Diaphragm breathing is the complete breath. Consciously change your breathing pattern. Use your diaphragm to breathe. Place one hand on your breastbone, feeling that it is raised, and put the other hand above your waist, feeling your diaphragm muscles moving up and down. Deep breathing with your diaphragm gives you complete breath. This is *how* you do your diaphragm breathing:

- Sit comfortably.
- Begin your slow exhalation through your nose.
- Contract your abdomen to empty your lungs.

- Begin your slow inhalation and simultaneously make your belly bulge out.
- While continuing your slow inhalation, now, slightly contract your abdomen and simultaneously lift your chest and hold.
- Continue your slow inhalation, and slowly raise your shoulders. This allows the air to enter fully into your lungs to attain the complete breath.
- Retain your breath and slightly raise your shoulders for a count of 5.
- Very slowly exhale the air. Your upper chest deflates first, and then your abdomen relaxes in.
- Repeat the process.

Learn to slowly prolong your breath, especially your exhalation. Relax your chest and diaphragm muscles, so that you can extend your exhalation, making your breathing out slightly longer and complete. To prolong your exhalation, count "one-and-two-and-three" as you breathe in and breathe out. Make sure that they become balanced. Once you have mastered that, then try to make your breathing out a little longer than your breathing in.

# APPENDIX C

# MINDFULNESS

Mindfulness is purposeful attention to the present moment. Practicing mindfulness is your path to the present moment. Anything you experience after coming into presence through mindfulness may become richer and more meaningful to you. This is how and why mindfulness can give you better health and greater happiness. In mindfulness, you recognize your thoughts as they occur, but you pay nonjudgmental attention to them; in other words, they neither distract nor disturb you, and you just observe them, like watching a movie about you unfolding before your very eyes.

If you are mindful of what your body and your mind are experiencing in the present moment, you will soon learn to become mindful of others, which is the beginning of compassion and loving-kindness—a quality that enriches life. If you are mindful of others, you will also become mindful of everything else in life, such as your breathing and your eating. Breathing comes so natural that many of us are not mindful of how we breathe, so many of us do not breathe right. As a result of incorrect breathing, we get less oxygen to our lungs, cells, and organs, and thus leading to health deterioration. Likewise, eating becomes second nature to us that many of us are no longer mindful of the eating process: we simply shuffle and stuff food into our mouths, mindless of chewing and digesting the food we are eating. Indeed, in our daily routines, there are so many things that we are mindless about, because we have taken them for granted. Mindfulness is re-directing our attention to what we are doing at the present moment to re-establish the vital link between the body and the mind.

## Mindfulness Walking

Walking is one of the best exercises. Be mindful of your walking: the walk must be brisk with full awareness and deep concentration of the mind. Very often, we are so caught up with our destination that we put our feet into automatic pilot, while our minds drift from one thought to another. To stop our rambling thoughts, we must train our minds to concentrate through mindfulness while we are walking briskly.

Mindfulness walking requires you to pay full attention to what you are doing, to notice the movement of your limbs, the shifting of your body weight as you move your right and left foot. Mindfulness walking gives you an opportunity to quiet your mind, to practice subliminal messages, to enhance your mental concentration.

Here is an example of how you can walk with mindfulness:

You can choose the first two verses from the famous **Psalm 23: "The Lord is my Shepherd. I shall not want."** Repeat each syllable in your mind with each foot as you walk step by step, one step at a time. Always begin with your right foot, and then followed by your left foot; continue your steps following each syllable with the corresponding right or left foot:

"The Lord is my She-pherd. I shall not want"
**R    L    R L    R    L    R L    R    L**

You always begin the first word with the right foot. So, if you have to begin the first word with the left foot instead, then you know you have messed up somewhere; in other words, you mind must have wandered off. When that happens, start all over again with your right foot first, followed by your left foot. You may be very surprised that within a 10 to 20 minute walk you might have messed up the sequence and coordination several times, because your mind did not concentrate enough.

You can choose any phrase other than the above.

## Meditation

Meditation is thinking about one thing at a time. Simple as it may seem, this requires practice and discipline. According to **St. Theresa of Avila**, the mind is like an unbridled horse wandering where it will, and your role is to train the horse, and gently and lovingly bring it back to the right course.

Meditation is training your mental attention to sharpen your awareness of what is going on in your mind. Once you see clearly what is going on in the present moment, you can then choose to ignore or to act upon what you are seeing through your mind.

## *Meditation Basics*

To meditate, you must get into the right frame of mind; that is, you must learn some meditation basics in order to know *how* to meditate effectively:

- You must be in a quiet environment conducive to meditation.
- Your body must be comfortable and still, and very relaxed.
- Your breathing must be right: inhale and exhale softly and slowly, preferably in a rhythm.
- Your mind must be focused, staying in the present moment, as much as possible.
- You must not expect anything to happen during the meditation session. You must always practice with consistency and persistence.

## How to Meditate

Find a quiet place where you can remain undisturbed for 10 to 30 minutes. To set the environment for meditation, you may want to have some scent from flowers or incense, or even some soothing music (meditation MP3) to enhance your senses. Of course, you can meditate without them; it is just an option, not a requirement.

Find time to practice meditation. Regularity holds the key to success in meditation. Do not meditate only when you feel like it. Find some quiet time to yourself everyday. The ideal time to meditate is before retiring to bed; in that way, your mind can review what has happened during the day—what you have said and done—and let go of everything. After all, meditation is about letting go of the past and future thoughts.

Correct posture is important. Firstly, your body must be erect: this induces correct breathing, which can bring all your internal energies into a state of harmony. Therefore, do not lean back on anything. If you find that your neck is too week and your spine cannot support your body, then rest your back on a hard surface initially; but the ultimate goal is to sit erect without your back touching anything.

You can sit cross-legged on the floor. Alternatively, you can sit comfortably on a chair (not a sofa), with your thighs at right angles to your spine, your hands on your thighs, your feet resting firmly on the floor, and your shoulders relaxed. In short, just sit "tall" and erect.

Begin meditation with your breathing. Your breathing is an indicator of your stress level: if you are unduly stressed, your breathing becomes thick and gasping. Breathing right is your conscious control of stress. When you feel stressed, consciously change your breathing pace to undo the stress.

Gently close your eyes, or you can fix your eyes on an object.

As you begin your meditation, you will find that your first thought does not come to your mind right away. When it finally comes, do not dismiss it. Instead, consciously focus on your breathing. That thought will then slowly disappear. After a while, another thought or the same thought may come up to your mind. Again, do not consciously dismiss it; re-focus on your breathing. With more practice, you will find that within a 10-minute time frame, fewer and fewer thoughts will crop up in your mind because your mind has stayed in the present moment for a longer period. The fewer thoughts you have, the more relaxed you become. Then, one day, you may suddenly find that you have stepped into a different world with total tranquility and clarity of thinking—even though it may last but a very brief moment. That euphoric sensation is nondescript. Once you have attained that inexplicable and transformative state of mind, you will want to continue practicing meditation everyday. But don't expect that transcendental state will come any time soon; the more you anticipate it, the longer it will take you to attain that state of mind. Just consistently and patiently practice meditation everyday.

Meditation is life-changing, especially in the golden years. Meditation may change *how* you look at yourself and your depression.

# APPENDIX D

## ABOUT THE AUTHOR

**About Stephen Lau**

http://www.stephencmlau.com

**Books by Stephen Lau:**

http://www.booksbystephenlau.com

**Stephen Lau's Related Blogs:**

http://reflectionsofstephenlau.blogspot.com
http://increase-mind-power.blogspot.com
http://tao-wisdom-and-biblical-isdom.blogspot.com
http://the-way-through-depression.blogspot.com

**Stephen Lau's Related Sites:**

http://www.health-and-wisdom-tips.com
http://www.wisdominliving.com

**Contact:**

stephencmlau@gmail.com